Bra Wars

Bra Wars

The Struggle Against Decency

Marie Audemard

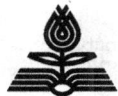

PETER LANG

Oxford - Berlin - Bruxelles - Chennai - Lausanne - New York

Bibliographic information published by the Deutsche Nationalbibliothek.
The German National Library lists this publication in the German National Bibliography;
detailed bibliographic data is available on the Internet at http://dnb.d-nb.de.

A catalogue record for this book is available from the British Library.

Library of Congress Cataloging-in-Publication Data

Names: Audemard, Marie, 1999- author.
Title: Bra wars : the struggle against decency / Marie Audemard.
Description: Oxford ; New York : Peter Lang, 2024. | Includes
   bibliographical references and index.
Identifiers: LCCN 2023052172 (print) | LCCN 2023052173 (ebook) |
   ISBN 9781803741451 (paperback) | ISBN 9781803741468 (ebook) |
   ISBN 9781803741475 (epub)
Subjects: LCSH: Clothing and dress—Symbolic aspects. | Brassieres—Social
   aspects. | Breast—Social aspects. | Body image in women—Public
   opinion. | Indecent exposure—Philosophy.
Classification: LCC GT2073 .A925 2024 (print) | LCC GT2073 (ebook) | DDC
   391.4/23—dc23/eng/20240131
LC record available at https://lccn.loc.gov/2023052172
LC ebook record available at https://lccn.loc.gov/2023052173

Cover image: Cover illustration copyrights: Jasmine Menear.
Cover design by Peter Lang Group AG

ISBN 978-1-80374-145-1 (print)
ISBN 978-1-80374-146-8 (ePDF)
ISBN 978-1-80374-147-5 (ePub)
DOI 10.3726/b20742

© 2024 Peter Lang Group AG, Lausanne
Published by Peter Lang Ltd, Oxford, United Kingdom
info@peterlang.com – www.peterlang.com

This publication has been peer reviewed.

If you aren't outraged,
you aren't paying attention

Contents

Figures

Acknowledgements

This project has been an essential part of my academic and personal journey and would not have been manageable without these fantastic people. First, thank you to my supervisor, Emma Rees, who answered every question I had – believe me, there were a lot of them – and motivated me. I am equally grateful to Louisa Yates, who provided many inspirational writing exercises during the Boot Camp and helped stimulate our creativity. I must also extend my thanks to Roger Hyde and Alex May, who spent so much time correcting my English and whose kind words always motivated me to keep going. Jasmine, thank you for putting so much work into this beautiful cover; you are so talented and brought it to life. A special mention goes to my wonderful editor, Laurel Plapp. Your guidance not only made my first experience with publishing enjoyable but also taught me so much.

Thank you to all my friends and family who listened to me talk about this project for hours and reassured me every time I got stressed – a special shoutout to Brett who probably spent hours motivating me on the low days. To Mum, Tatiana, and Mica, thank you for answering all the calls and helping me figure out the answers when I didn't know what to think. I am so grateful for you. To all my friends, your involvement and shared excitement for this project mean the world to me. Finally, thank you more specifically to my parents and brother, who supported me through my ongoing fight against misogyny. Thank you for spending years making our household a safe space so I could be myself.

Introduction

She should *hide* her breasts.
Why is she trying so hard to *attract* men?
Her nipples are showing; that's so *indecent*.
She's such a *prick-tease*. She's begging to be *raped*.

Upsetting, isn't it? Hearing these comments is as disturbing as reading in the news that 20% of French people still believe that visible nipples could justify men assaulting women.[1] Bras have always been a subject of debate, used to entice, support, eroticise, or only worn for comfort. Still, women's breasts have rarely been free from the constraint of having to be moulded or padded. For decades, they have been considered sexual in Western countries and are now highly regulated body parts.[2] In this book, a central concept explored is 'decency,' which is frequently linked to femininity and nudity.[3] It is a term often used in hushed tones when people observe a woman revealing too much skin. 'Decency' serves as the foundation for defining which parts of women's bodies are deemed acceptable to expose.

While dress codes apply to all genders, there have been, historically, many more concerns and control over female clothing choices.[4] In other words, 'decency' regulates women to ensure they display their bodies without causing scandal.[5] You have undoubtedly heard it at least once: 'What will people think if she wears that? That *she doesn't respect herself.*' You might even have said it yourself or looked at your reflection in the mirror and thought, 'I should get changed; people will think I am a slut.' Yet, what you did not know that day is here; these thoughts were the product of decency norms. They are repeated so often in women's environments that they infiltrate how we think, perceive, act, and judge.

Researchers have worked on how breasts or lingerie became sexual, but none truly worked on the relationship between the two. Therefore, my research aims to enlarge the scope of knowledge in gender studies on this

matter. Moreover, my research is based in France, which is a country where
gender studies are not entirely accepted yet.[6] France is often described as
a country with a liberal attitude towards sexuality and nudity, sometimes
perceived as an 'erotic' nation.[7] This led me to delve into the question of
whether its reputation as a 'sexually liberated' country truly embodies
absolute freedom or if it is merely a façade concealing the continued oppression and objectification of women. This research also aims to raise
awareness of women's oppression through underwear. My work might help
people be more aware of their own internalised decency – see below – and,
therefore, allow women's bodies to be less regulated. Although I focus on
French women, the scope of this book goes beyond France. As you read
through these pages, you may recognise some of the experiences I describe
and think, 'Yes, I've felt that too.' Sadly, the truth is that most women in
Western countries, and many more across the world, have encountered the
decency norms that I address in this book – albeit with some variations.
This global issue affects patriarchal societies everywhere, so even if you are
not French or particularly interested in French culture, I believe you will
find this book relevant and relatable.

       In the following chapters, you will discover how clothes can simultan-
eously reveal and conceal. Yet, women are expected to magically strike the
perfect balance between decency and attractiveness. By the end, I will have
given you the answer to one question: how do bras participate in making
breasts – especially nipples – socially indecent?

       Why nipples, in particular? Because I still hear my girlfriends shout
across the room while they get ready, 'I can't wear that; people can see my
nipples.' Because since I can remember, people have always commented
on when my nipples were showing. And because seamless bras and nipple
covers have become the default tools to hide this part of the breast. While
writing this book, I graduated with my Master's in Gender Studies. I ordered
a beautiful dress for the big day and got a 'surprise gift' with it. I spent days
wondering what it would be: a cute necklace, a bracelet or maybe some
earrings I saw on the website? It finally arrived, and what an ironic surprise
it was to find two nipple covers next to my dress. This anecdote alone can
answer the question of why talking about nipples is essential – because
even a random dress shop feels the need to remind me that I cannot wear

my dress without hiding them. Nipples are now associated with showing the natural shape of the breasts and, therefore, with indecency.

I introduce in this project the concept of *internalised decency* developed based on all the reading and interviews I have done. *Internalised decency* can result from many situations, including when women grow up hearing that they are not meant to display their bodies or specific body parts. In the case of the women I interviewed, almost all internalised decency rules because of comments from people around them, peer pressure, advertisements, or books. All these were created because of a broader context you will discover in this book. If you are already wondering why I chose to use the word 'decency' instead of 'modesty' since these two might nearly refer to the same thing, here is my explanation. The concept of the 'modesty cult' described in Victoria Bateman's book *Naked Feminism* perfectly fits my argument, and what I call 'indecency' here is directly linked to it. However, I chose to use a different word for two reasons. First, to genuinely depict how French people mean it. I grew up in France and never heard people say, 'That's so immodest' – 'immodeste' in French. However, I heard people say, 'That's so indecent' and subconsciously dissimulate the modesty cult behind this word. 'Indecency' is the word I have heard from my interviewees, friends, family, or classmates when discussing a woman not following social norms. The second reason is that the notion of 'modesty' regulates women's bodies and forces them to hide. However, for a few decades, Western societies have not only continued to pressure women to conceal their breasts, but they also started forcing them to be 'enticing' in the right way. Women in Western countries, such as France, must navigate a delicate balance to be considered attractive and respectable. Consequently, as these new 'rules' blend modesty with over-sexualisation, I have chosen to refer to them as 'decency norms' and 'internalised decency'.

This project involves a blend of autoethnography and individual interviews, rooted in the principles of intersectional standpoint epistemology. By considering multiple variables – in this case, gender and age – this study aims to incorporate diverse perspectives. Notably, some participants grew up in the decade following the sexual revolution of 1968, making these variables particularly relevant for analysis.

You will meet in this book ten women who agreed to talk about their relationship with their breasts: Noa (19), Éléana (18), Tara (23), Emma (30), Lucie (31), Julia (38), Clara (41), Sarah (50), Romane (51) and Andréa (55).[8] All of them live in Paris and create a beautiful discussion around indecency. Among them, Tara, Clara, Emma, and Noa describe themselves as large-breasted, which gives them different experiences from the rest of the women. Not all of the large-breasted women I interviewed needed to wear a bra for support. Noa did not wear one at all unless she felt pressured to 'correct her sagging breasts,' as she was self-conscious and concerned about social acceptance. Emma wore a bra every day when going out but looked forward to taking it off as soon as she got home, knowing that no one could sexualise her there. Thus, her bra was not needed for support. Tara and Clara, on the other hand, both needed bras for support, but they also acknowledged the sexual dimension that influenced their decision to wear them. When asked if she would still wear a bra if she didn't need it for support, Tara said she probably would because she disliked her nipples being visible. Since my book focuses on 'how conditioned women are to wear bras to be decent' rather than 'why women are wearing bras,' I will not cover the need for support among large-breasted women. Instead, I will analyse how large-breasted women, more than other the other women I interviewed, are sexualised, and conditioned to be perceived as decent.

This topic can also spark a discussion on different ethnicities and their relationship with bras. As I delve into the impact of colonialism within this context, it's important to acknowledge that my research primarily includes participants who are white, with only one out of ten interviewees being a Person of Colour. This demographic composition can indeed shape how norms and expectations are perceived. Given the limited representation of People of Colour in my study, drawing comprehensive conclusions on the specific influences of colonialism and racial dynamics on views of bras may be challenging. However, it is crucial to emphasise that participant ethnicity can significantly influence perceptions and experiences, even in discussions of undergarments.

To my knowledge, no research has been conducted on the specific relationship between ethnicities and bras in France yet. Nonetheless, several researchers have delved into the question of race and women's sexualisation in Western countries, such as the United States. For example, the book *Ain't I a Beauty Queen?*[9] by Maxine Leeds Craig thoroughly explores the intricate relationship between beauty, race, and power within American society, with a particular focus on the experiences of Black women. Craig analyses the historical construction and manipulation of beauty ideals, revealing how they have been used to marginalise Black women, perpetuate racial stereotypes, and uphold Eurocentric beauty standards. Additionally, Shayne Lee's work, *Erotic Revolutionaries: Black Women, Sexuality, and Popular Culture,*[10] complements this argument by shedding light on the often overlooked intersections of race, gender, and sexuality that Black women have confronted throughout history. The book emphasises how Black women have navigated and challenged societal norms and stereotypes related to their sexuality, making significant contributions to shaping popular culture in areas like music, film, literature, and various media forms. However, the link between ethnicity and bra-wearing would benefit from exploration by other scholars in the future.

In a world where breasts are often viewed as sexual objects, it's essential to understand how we got here. In the first chapter, we delve into how women's breasts became sexualised and lingerie's role in the past centuries. We also uncover the influence of religion and economic interests in shaping societal expectations around women's bodies, leading to the widespread belief that women should hide their breasts.

Moving on to the second chapter, we take a closer look at French women living in Paris and their complex relationship with breast coverage. We explore how capitalism and patriarchy are intertwined in shaping these women's decisions and how they struggle with the tension between private versus public presentation.

Chapter 3 examines the dichotomy between online and offline decency norms. We explore the role that people's perceptions of what is considered appropriate behaviour play in hypersexualisation.

Finally, in Chapter 4, we explore the impact of peers, family, and mothers' pressure on their daughters regarding sexualisation. We examine how patterns repeat themselves from generation to generation and how parents often unknowingly pass on their own beliefs and biases.

I believe we can only work towards creating a more equal world by understanding where the oppression comes from. Although this book might not change the way Western societies perceive and sexualise women's bodies, I hope it can help you feel better about your own and challenge the regulations that are imposed upon it. How did we feel pressured to wear something in the first place? Why do we continue to wear it even though we can't wait to take it off? I hope that this book will answer your questions …
… and inspire you to ask some more.

The making of the indecent breast

Do not be too sexy but still pleasant to look at, please.
– Judith Lussier, *Un symbole d'oppression*

When I mention how sexualised bras are in conversations, people often respond that women might wear them mainly for support, not because it has been imposed on them. And they are right. There have been times when women used bras to support and make their daily lives easier. Similarly, some women still wear them purely for comfort nowadays, and breast size plays a massive part in whether a woman can live a braless lifestyle. However, no matter your breast size and why you choose to wear underwear, breasts, and bras have a sexual dimension and are socially regulated in many cultures worldwide. And this cannot be ignored.

Before delving into breast-specific concerns, it is essential to provide context on how modesty norms have regulated women's bodies for centuries. Western cultures have traditionally required women to conceal their bodies entirely due to the modesty cult. In her book, Victoria Bateman explains that various factors could have led to the regulation of women's bodies. While we will explore the influence of religion and economic interests, it is vital to note how inherently oppressive patriarchal societies are towards women's bodies because of how they function. Like almost every other country, France operates under a patriarchal system where women give birth to children that continue the man's lineage.[1] However, since men could not be sure if the child was theirs, they found a solution: regulating women's bodies. Heterosexual men began controlling women's dress, behaviour, and movement, hoping to prevent them from having sex with other men.[2] Researcher Alice Evans explains that 'the entire sense of honour and shame in a patrilineal society is bound up to the sexual propriety of women. Therefore, the whole society is organised around removing any and all doubt about the virginity of unmarried women and the fidelity of wives.'[3] And that, for example, by forbidding them to wear anything that could draw attention to their bodies for centuries.

1/ From nurturing to sexual

From 3000 BCE until the twentieth century, many European people chose to breastfeed as the best way to feed their babies, leading to the creation of wet nurses. These women could be paid to feed babies when the mother could not provide for hers, for example, because she was ill or unable to produce milk.[4] However, France, along with other Western countries, used enslaved women from the Global South to breastfeed the children of their 'owners'. These women would often be separated from their own children for extended periods.[5] During the eighteenth century in France, about 80% of children were wet nursed.[6] In Europe, royal families would almost systematically employ wet nurses because breastfeeding was perceived as 'too common' to be undertaken by royal women.[7] Because the task of feeding a baby was visible, breasts became a powerful symbol of maternity. Breastfeeding was an increasing phenom-enon during the French Revolution of 1789.[8] In 1792, the French emblem, Marianne – a woman with bare breasts – became the allegory of the re-public. She was the official representation of freedom, equality, and fra-ternity values. Therefore, breastfeeding in public became how women expressed their support for the republic – French women only obtained the right to vote in 1945 (see Figure 1).

French people still question Marianne's bare breasts nowadays. How could the French Republic symbol be a naked woman when 69% of French women aged under 25 years old say they cannot go out without a bra as they fear their nipples being visible?[9] Marianne was created in a context where breasts were associated with motherhood and a way for women

Figure 1: Eugène Delacroix, *La liberté guidant le peuple*, 1930. Commonly used to
represent Marianne.

to be involved in politics. This way, she was a maternal symbol of the republic, not a woman breaking free. In a debate about Marianne being
bare-breasted, French minister Manuel Valls said, 'Marianne has a naked
breast because she is feeding the people, she is not veiled, because she is
free! That is the republic.'[10]

   It is tempting to infer that women had been allowed to show their
breasts as they were almost socially required to breastfeed; however, this is
not the case. First, women were rarely welcome in public spaces like cafes
in the eighteenth and nineteenth centuries. 'Public' for them meant private
places with some people in the same room.[11] Their dresses were also designed
so they had a secret part allowing them to breastfeed without showing
the entirety of their breasts. Usually, there would be slits cut around the
breast part of the bodice.[12] Even before the breast was perceived as sexual,

women's bodies were not allowed to be displayed because of the modesty cult already in place and mainly regulated by Christianity. If breasts were still considered primarily nurturing for a bit after the French Revolution, Sigmund Freud's theories and capitalism were about to change that.

Sigmund Freud and child-mother sexuality

Freud was one of the most prominent figures who shifted the perception of breasts from being 'maternal' to 'sexual' due to his theories.[13] He wrote about breasts at the end of the nineteenth century and the beginning of the twentieth century, and these concepts significantly transformed breastfeeding culture and social norms.[14] Freud argued that 'the key to sexuality is to be found between parents and child,' and he added that suckling on the nipples creates the child's libido, which would explain why heterosexual men are fascinated with women's breasts.[15] According to him, children associate the comfort of their mother with the breast. So, when a boy eventually needs to stop sucking on his mother, he will spend the rest of his life trying to fill the gap, resulting in an obsession with breasts.[16] By theorising that a boy's development involves a crucial stage of desiring his mother, Freud contributed to the sexualisation of women's bodies in the psychoanalytic framework. This sexualisation has broader implications for gender relations and power dynamics. By reducing women to objects of male desire, the sexualisation of women's bodies reinforces traditional patriarchal norms, which can lead to the objectification and marginalisation of women, reducing their agency and personhood.[17] Freud's portrayal of breastfeeding as a potential sexual activity between a child and their mother had far-reaching consequences. It led to shifts in social norms, associating breasts more with sexuality than with their maternal function. The book *Cultural History of the Breast* explains how the social notions of 'possession' and 'privacy' have been associated with breasts due to this shift:

> Breastfeeding offers reciprocal pleasures between the giver and the receiver – a fact
> that in past times was openly acknowledged in medical texts and other documents but

which today has become associated with considerable taboo. It is safe to assume that this is because mother-infant sensuality threatens the heterosexual conjugal bond.[18]

Freud also wrote theories on the 'fight' between the son and the father to win the mother's breasts.[19] He explained how, to him, the jealousy felt by the boy realising that his mother was 'already taken' was the initial stage of the long Oedipal father/son fight. This struggle would supposedly last until the son eventually regulates his own needs and finds another woman to fill this sexual gap. However, Freud's work has since been viewed as highly heteronormative and misogynistic.

In her book *Psychoanalysis and Feminism*, Juliet Mitchell provides a nuanced perspective on Freud's theories, arguing that psychoanalysis is a description of patriarchy's workings rather than an endorsement of it.[20] Mitchell's analysis helps shed light on the conflicted nature of Freud's ideas and their impact on societal perceptions. She argues that Freud's theories tend to downplay and marginalise women's experiences and subjectivity. Notably, the Oedipus complex, in its original formulation, was centred around the male experience, leaving little room for the complexities of female development. However, it's worth noting that Mitchell's argument is not a direct contradiction but rather an exploration of how Freud's work both describes patriarchy and, inadvertently, diminishes women's subjectivity. This exclusion of the female perspective results in a limited understanding of women's roles and desires, further reinforcing traditional gender stereotypes and societal expectations. Unfortunately, Freud's views transformed how women's breasts were perceived and allowed heterosexual men to control women's bodies even more.

How capitalism created a new market out of breasts

At the same time, bottle feeding arrived in the US around 1930, during the Great Depression, as the country sought to boost consumption and emerge from the economic crisis.[21] This new era of industrialisation transformed how women's breasts were socially perceived.[22] Women quickly became direct victims of capitalism and patriarchy as Western countries marketed bottles, industrial milk, and other tools to help them feed their babies more efficiently, allowing them to focus on household chores. The goal was also to make baby feeding more 'glamourous'.[23] Women were freed from the exhausting task of feeding their babies themselves but oppressed in new and different ways.

As advertisements claimed that bottle feeding was a better option than breastfeeding, breasts slowly became sexualised by and for the male gaze. Pitts-Taylor explains that 'women's breasts were then free from the drudgery of their functional role and turned instead into luxury items for the entertainment and consumption of the heterosexual male'.[24] Technological, historical, and economic changes increased the sexualisation of women's breasts, primarily due to how common pornography became. In addition, globalisation exported Western values to every part of the globe, leading many countries to also sexualise women's breasts.[25] Breasts were no longer just a way to feed babies; they were visually pleasing body parts owned by heterosexual men. The perfect example was during the Second World War when American magazines began featuring a brand-new concept: the 'Pin-up' girl.[26] Magazines like *Esquire* portrayed these women as large-breasted with a tiny waist and long legs, describing them as the 'perfect version of femininity'.[27] Soldiers received copies to 'lift their mood', making them hopeful of returning to the women waiting back home. This period marked the beginning of 'mammary madness',[28] where pin-up girls were ubiquitous, even illustrated on war bombs and aircraft. This sexualisation profoundly impacted the bodies of all women. During the colonial era, Western societies, including France, engaged in a pseudo-scientific and ethnographic exploration of the 'exotic' and 'primitive' world of the Global South.[29] Magazines like National Geographic played a significant role in shaping the colonial gaze, disseminating images that reinforced harmful stereotypes and objectified the women of these regions. These publications often depicted women from the Global South as hypersexualised, mysterious, and submissive figures, reinforcing the idea that they were exotic 'other' beings.[30] These images not only served as a form of visual entertainment for Western audiences but also justified the colonisation and exploitation of these regions. The colonial gaze stripped these women of their agency, culture, and identity, reducing them to mere objects of fascination and curiosity.

Since infant formula had been introduced and breasts hypersexualised, western opinion on breastfeeding quickly declined. This practice was discouraged in the media and perceived as only for lower classes of women as it was 'indecent'.[31] Simultaneously, wet nursing also became highly taboo, and the exposure of a now considered 'intimate' body part made people uncomfortable.[32] In 2023, breastfeeding in public in Europe remains a significant debate in each country as governments continue to discuss decency and breast visibility issues.[33] In France, breastfeeding in public is not officially forbidden, but many cases of assault – predominantly verbal – have been recorded and justified by 'indecency'.[34] Once again, social norms and rules prevent women from displaying *their* bodies based on what is considered 'respectable'.[35]

2/ Don't be a sl*t like Eve

Christianity, and specifically Catholicism, has long been the dominant religion in France significantly shaping various social norms, particularly those concerning women's bodies.[36] The concept of modesty, often associated with Christianity, has persisted over time and created what is known as the 'cult of modesty'.[37] This notion perpetuated the belief that women's bodies were inherently indecent and that men were helpless to control their sexual impulses.[38] To safeguard women's virtue, religious figures offered solutions, advocating for modest dress and a sense of invisibility. As a result, the Church laid the foundation for the decency norms that continue to pressure French women – as well as many women globally – to conform to certain standards of dress and behaviour. Despite the waning influence of the Church in modern European countries, including France, the lasting legacy of centuries of Christianity's impact and patriarchal structures has led to the internalisation of expectations regarding women's conduct, clothes and expression. Society now imposes standards of 'indecency', which, in reality, serve as veiled expressions of another form of modesty. This subtle influence continues to govern

women's bodies, albeit imperceptibly, perpetuating the ideals of decency
and modesty that have deep historical roots in Christianity.

Eve and Virgin Mary's stories as a standard for women

The first biblical story pushing Christians to demonise women and regulate their bodies was The Garden of Eden. According to the story, Eve
charmed Adam, causing him to sin by eating the apple from the Tree
of Life. Heterosexual men saw this as one of the reasons why women
should be repressed, dominated, and silenced, so they could not 'use their
charms' on men other than the one they 'belonged to'. Mati Meyer explains that from the fourth century, Eve was portrayed in a misogynistic
way and described as 'destructive to male rationality'.[39] Women were either portrayed as 'virginal goddesses' or 'evil temptresses' with no middle
ground.[40] Women were not individuals; they were the 'fall of all men'.

Eve was perceived as 'too tempting' for heterosexual men, like she
had been for Adam, pushing him to bite the apple. Being seen as a temp-
tress, she was considered a passive object of sexual desire for heterosexual
men. To keep their reputation safe, women should have avoided anything
resembling this story.

The Christian lifestyle of the Virgin Mary was another story holding
women to stringent standards. To be considered 'pure' and 'good', they were
expected to emulate Mary's lifestyle and strive to be the 'perfect Christian'
by embodying traits such as purity, submission, silence, and motherhood.[41]
However, despite some women being deemed 'pure and modest', their
submission to men and the demand for their bodies to remain quiet and
invisible persisted. As written in the Bible in 1 Timothy 2:9–15:

> I also want the women to dress modestly, with decency and propriety, adorning them-
> selves, not with elaborate hairstyles or gold or pearls or expensive clothes, but with
> good deeds appropriate for women who profess to worship God. A woman should
> learn in quietness and full submission. I do not permit a woman to teach or to as-
> sume authority over a man; she must be quiet. For Adam was formed first, then Eve.[42]

Virgin Mary was, however, frequently represented breastfeeding – called the *Madonna Lactans*, and therefore, showing her breasts. How was it respectable to do so when she was meant to be the 'perfect' Christian woman? First, artists mainly represented Mary's breasts in weird or un-recognisable shapes. That way, it did not go against the 'proximity created between nakedness and carnal lust ever since Adam and Eve ate the for-bidden fruit of the Garden of Eden'.[43] Second, Mary was perceived as a mother and not as 'tempting'; she was 'sanitised pornography'.[44] However, portraits of the Virgin Mary's breastfeeding were strongly discouraged after the sixteenth century as it was increasingly considered indecent.[45]

Purity culture and 'being a decent woman'

In the Middle Ages European societies, women's decency and compliance with purity culture made them 'respectable' and 'worthy'. First, the term 'purity culture' needs to be defined. Initially, this term referred to the American Evangelical Christian purity movement launched in the 1990s. However, purity culture is also centuries of religious and patriarchal heri-tage and is now a global social phenomenon intrinsically linked with modesty. You can see the impact of purity culture in many things that so-cialised humans do.[46] For example, when women are slut-shamed because they had sex with 'too many people' or when they are told they cannot wear a crop top. Most of the time, 'slut-shaming' and 'purity culture' play on the same team. For example, suppose a woman is considered a 'temp-tress'; she might be slut-shamed as a reminder to abide by decency norms. Purity culture is aimed at women. I could bet that you have probably never heard a man being told to dress 'decently' if they want to be 'the right type of guy'. Purity culture massively participates in making women internalise decency norms as it can make them think they must dress in the 'right way' to be respectable.

Since the story of the Garden of Eden, where Adam and Eve realised that they were naked and needed to dress up, various clothing items have been ruling people's lives – especially women's. During France's fourteenth and fifteenth centuries, clothing was the scale people used to assess if women were 'decent' or followed an 'immoral' lifestyle. However, 'decency' is linked to 'virginity' when it comes to women and must be preserved.[47] Marie De Rasse explains it perfectly: 'The woman exposing her body, entirely or partially, is indecent, not because of her nudity, but because she is tempting men.'[48] For this reason, they had to be covered.

The ancestor of the bra, the 'chemise', was the first clothing layer that women had to wear and needed to be invisible to men other than their husbands.[49] This chemise also had to be white, without any stain, as a symbol of purity and honour. Around 1850, a middle-class woman's sexual reputation was often her only way to exist in society and guarantee her 'material well-being and social standing through marriage'.[50] Therefore, specific actions, like wearing inappropriate clothes or arguing for women's rights, damaged their reputations and needed to be avoided and regulated. Christianity stopped being linked with the state in 1905 in France. As a general phenomenon in Europe, countries like the United Kingdom, France, and Germany – called the 'reformed West' – stopped being as religious as they used to be.[51] A lot has changed regarding social norms. Western women are now pressured to dress modestly and decently while staying attractive enough to the outside world and to their husbands through sexuality and lingerie in private. According to some religious figures, women's role is to keep men interested in the relationship through sex. A perfect example of this private/public dichotomy occurred in America in 2013 when former Southern Baptist minister Pat Robertson made comments on how women should continue to entice their partners by being sexy or would be to blame for marital problems if they did not.[52] As an answer, Kristen Rosser, a Christian blogger, wrote:

'Be modest.'

'Be beautiful.' 'Don't cause a man to stumble.' 'Don't let yourself go.'

Today, Christians are adept at holding, at the same time, attitudes that women should be outwardly beautiful/sexy and modest/sexually concealed. The shaming of Christian women for supposedly not staying attractive to their husbands is a prime example of the former - while, by contrast, Christian men remain nearly exempt from any teaching that they should try to stay attractive to their wives.[53]

Kristen's argument perfectly encapsulates the dichotomy that lay at the heart of the sexual revolution of 1968 in France, arising from centuries of inherited Christian regulation on women's bodies. Women were pressured to be seductive and sexual in private for their male partner and were expected to wear sexy lingerie or enhance their breasts.[54] However, they were unable to dress as they desired in public as it was deemed enticing and inappropriate to other men. Women fought against these expectations, striving to break free from the notion that they belonged to a man. On her website, Pastor and author Ruth Everhart published a post in response to articles about Mississippi Baptist Stewart-Allen Clark. Clark claimed that women were responsible for what their husbands looked at and should not give them a reason to stray.[55] Everhart denounces the pressure put on women by the church to not 'tempt' men while being enticing:

> Women are responsible for their husband's lustful leering at other women. Therefore, they must be slim and attractive. Women are responsible when men other than their husbands lustfully gaze upon them. Therefore, they must dress modestly. In short, women are responsible for all the actions that follow when a man lustfully leers. Lustful leering is his God-given right because 'that's how God made him'. (…) Ask any women who grew up in church culture, and I guarantee that she has heard that she is responsible for the male eyes that rest upon her. When I was growing up, I was told that I needed to mind the length of my hem and the width of my shoulder straps because 'boys are visual'. Glimpsing a sliver too much of my skin would cause boys to sin, and that would be my fault.[56]

Through all these testimonies, it is clear that the modesty cult described in Marie de Rasse's study is still prevalent today. In the Middle Ages, Christianity led French society to believe that an honest woman should not show her chest – or any other part of her body. If she did, she would be considered immodest – therefore indecent – as she would expose herself to men's gaze.[57] Centuries later, some parts of women's bodies were slowly liberated from the modesty cult in Western countries like France. Legs started showing, but some body parts like breasts were considered sexual and had to stay hidden; they had already been reclaimed by heterosexual men.

In the context of modern-day France, the concept of women's modesty continues to evolve, with additional layers influenced by various cultural and religious perspectives. One such influence is the presence of Islamic traditions, which have introduced a distinct dimension to the discourse surrounding modesty. For many Muslim women, modesty holds a significant place within their religious beliefs and cultural practices.[58] Just as historical Christian norms shaped ideas of decency, Islamic teachings emphasise the importance of modest dress and behaviour as a means of upholding personal and communal values. The practice of hijab, a traditional head covering, stands as a visible representation of modesty for Muslim women, conveying not only their dedication to faith but also their commitment to self-respect and humility.[59] Yet, this expression of modesty has sparked contemporary discussions within French society, generating debates that extend beyond clothing to matters of integration, diversity, and the boundaries of secularism.[60] The clash of differing perceptions on modesty highlights the intricate interplay of beliefs and cultural backgrounds in the ongoing narrative of societal norms and women's autonomy. It becomes evident that the concept of modesty is a living, breathing entity that intertwines religious, social, and personal values.

3/ A brief history of bras

For centuries, women have worn various forms of underwear, each with their own unique shape and style. But no matter the form they take, they all share one thing in common: they have been used to oppress them. Ironically, women have also used bras as a tool to break free from societal constraints at times. One thing is for sure, the bra is a complex symbol imbued with erotic fetishism on one hand and a taboo-first layer meant to conceal the naked body on the other.[61] From needing to be totally erased to being decently displayed to be considered attractive, here is how heterosexual men changed the rules of the modesty game when it could benefit them.

Corsets

This undergarment was the star of the show in Europe until the twentieth century. However, its popularity declined, especially after the French couturier Paul Poiret created the first corsetless dress in 1908. By the end of the nineteenth century, women questioned the corset's use, but manufacturers paid scientists to prove that they should still wear them.[62] The Tango dance craze was also popular at the time, and women removed their corsets to dance freely. Quickly, they started rejecting Victorian morals and fashion styles associated with them as it restricted their movements. Women wanted to go to school, exercise, work, or participate in leisure activities, which was impossible with a corset and thus began their emancipation from this underwear.[63] Simone de Beauvoir described corsets in her book *The Second Sex* as 'the rules of property'. Not able to move, women would then 'present the inert and passive qualities of an object' and be men's properties.[64] Manufacturers created new dance corsets to prevent losing the market, not to 'end women's desire for fashion change, but to contain it'.[65] However, traditional corsets regained popularity after the Second World War as populations became nostalgic for their pre-war environment. Before, gender differentiation was more apparent, and women were subordinate to heterosexual men while being 'respectable' and 'desirable' to their husbands. As being a man was considered the norm, women's clothing had to make their differences visible. This was achieved by emphasising the breasts, waist, bottom, and hips.[66]

Global fashion and mass media emerged with industrialisation. As more countries became aware of what was happening around them, social norms started to expand, regulating women's clothing globally.[67] France was a significant influence in terms of fashion because of the bourgeoisie. Paris was perceived as the world's fashion capital because of brands like Louis Vuitton and Christian Dior. As brassieres slowly became more common, French women stopped wearing corsets in the 1930s.

Brassieres

Brassieres arrived in France at the beginning of the twentieth century, thanks to a French feminist called Herminie Cadolle, who introduced the 'Corselet-gorge' to the universal exhibition in Paris (see Figure 2).[68]

As this invention was much more freeing than the corset, it was perceived as a liberation for women and their ability to move. However, in 1920, women's beauty standards focused on making their breasts as flat as possible. Some researchers argue this may have been due to women fighting for gender equality, suffrage, work, and a desire for a more androgynous look. Yet, other researchers who conducted more critical analysis see it as an infantilisation of women's bodies and pressure to look as youthful as teenage girls.[69]

By the end of the 1920s, brassieres began to lift the breasts, with manufacturers promoting this uplift as 'the way to solve the damages caused by breast binding', which some women used to flatten their breasts.[70] Jill Fields explains that uplift became associated with the 1920s preoccupation with the look of youth and the emerging 1930s trend towards restoring the 'womanly figure'.[71] Before 1930, manufacturers made brassieres with

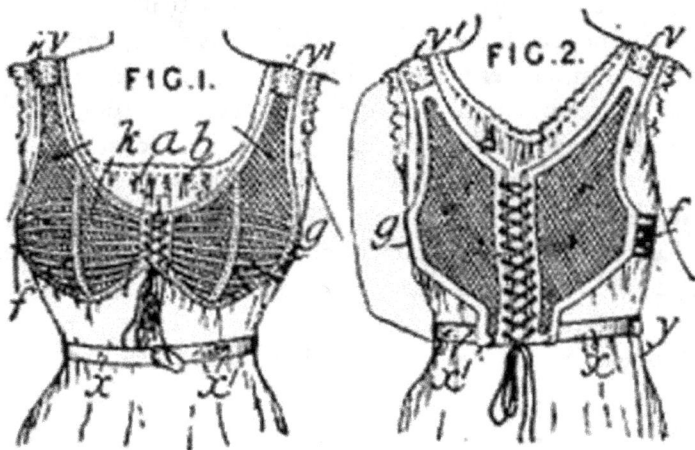

Figure 2: 'Corselet-gorge' by Herminie Cadolle.

a pointed cup shape called the 'pointed French effect'. It was considered sophisticated for a while until fashion rules changed. Women were expected to stop wearing the pointed cups as they were 'calling attention to the chest', which was considered vulgar. Instead, the round cups were perceived as more conservative and appropriate, as well as the new youthful look.[72] This time, the latest version of 'womanliness' involved mature and childlike appearance elements. Still, it pushed women to transform their natural bodies to fit a norm.

By the end of the 1930s, lifted breasts had become the norm, and manufacturers introduced seamless brassieres on the market as a way for women to look 'natural and feminine'.[73] The goal was to make breasts invisible but uplift the chest, which eventually redefined what a 'natural' breast looked like.[74] Brassieres sold so quickly that gradual breast cup sizes were introduced in the 1930s. Making the separation between the breasts noticeable became necessary, as it looked more youthful while still being 'feminine'. The importance of restoring the womanly figure became more evident after the Second World War when men returned home, and women had been doing the tasks typically assigned to men. Gender differentiation became too blurry for the patriarchy, and women had to make their upper bodies look more 'feminine' again.[75] The sexualisation of women's upper body parts happened after images of pin-up women – large-breasted, long legs and a tiny waist – had been used to boost the morale of soldiers fighting in the war. Jill Fields adds that 'large breasts enhance a woman's ability to attract male desire because they symbolise a haven of maternal nurturing and are appealing fetish objects in themselves'.[76] Therefore, wearing push-up bras and looking like a pin-up girl became ideal for women in that period.

Current bra uses

In 1960, feminists associated bras with oppression, so getting rid of them was one of their main ways of contesting the prevailing social norms during the sexual revolution of May 1968. Most women who continued to wear bras chose them primarily for comfort and avoided wearing ones considered 'sexy'.[77] After the revolution, going topless became common in France, especially on the beach, and was perceived worldwide as a feminist act for liberation. Women also demanded lighter and less padded bras, which would reveal more natural breasts regardless of whether it was going against the 'rules' or was deemed indecent.[78] Yet, in 2022, being topless has become taboo again. More than 57% of women aged 18 to 30 agree with being topless in their garden, whereas only 24% agree to be topless on the beach.[79] Though, some 60-year-old women and older who fought during the sexual revolution still go topless. The decreasing number of women doing so is due to the over-sexualisation of women's bodies, the persistent modesty cult, and the glamorisation of bras as sexual objects in the 1990s.[80] The *Wonderbra* ad, which reads 'Hello boys' next to a woman in underwear, perfectly illustrates the sexual connotation of breasts. However, the advert became controversial as it displayed women as passive objects of the male gaze. Later, *Wonderbra* unsuccessfully tried to switch the slogan to 'Hello me' to promote women's self-empowerment, but it was heavily criticised for being insincere.[81]

The creation of the *Victoria's Secret* brand was also a significant turning point in the sexualisation of women's bodies. The 'angels' of the brand were ultra-skinny, defined, and tall, representing an unrealistic body ideal for the 'average' woman.[82] Boudoir photography also became popular. Recently, bras have been reinvented many times, allowing women to wear them in any way possible to ensure they keep buying them.[83] While corsets and bras can support women with their daily tasks, they have also been used to oppress them or make their breasts visible only when heterosexual men want to look at them – in pornography or private settings, for example. An article in the media called *Métro* explains that bras are thought to prevent women from distracting men by flattening their nipples.[84] This also reinforces the 'high and round' beauty standards that govern breasts. As the article rightly concludes: 'The bra perfectly illustrates the very restrained spectrum of the female ideal: "Do not be too sexy but still pleasant to look at, please."'

Conclusion

At times, bras have been used to liberate women from corsets and integrate them slowly into society, sports, and work. Yet, it is also a gilded cage, socially oppressing women as it became a requirement to hide their breasts and nipples to be considered decent. The modesty cult has historically regulated women's bodies and continues to do so. Breasts were deemed appropriate to be 'publicly' visible when perceived as primarily maternal, but as soon as they started being seen as sexual, they had to be hidden to avoid tempting heterosexual men – except when looking at breasts would be pleasurable for them, of course. Breasts are still considered indecent, but women are now pressured to display them correctly to be socially attractive. Yet, the question remains: *what makes women internalise these expectations?*

CHAPTER 2

Why are you so provocative?

> It's her dream, of course. To be admired and desired by men.
> – Antoine in Emily in Paris

Since I can remember, I have always hated the word 'indecent'. Growing up with a Christian mother who had strict and conservative parents, she used to ask me to change my outfit before leaving for school because it was 'inappropriate' – some shorts and a top. I don't blame her; she has undergone the same 'moulding' process as most women on earth, and getting out of it is difficult. Yet, the words *inappropriate* and *indecent* stuck with me for years before I officially started my internal battle against them.

In 2018, I stopped wearing the bra during an internship in Paris. I wear a B cup and I never felt the need to wear one for support. As I come from the south of France, where everything is more 'traditional' than in the capital, I had always felt pressured to wear one – whether it was because I had been trained to see my breasts as unattractive without them being lifted, or because I knew my nipples weren't supposed to show. One day, I remember watching an American 24-year-old influencer on Instagram saying that she had bought her first bra and did not find it comfortable, so she would not be wearing one again. She explained that she never felt the need to as no one in her family did and that, up to that point, no one noticed this in her pictures. This influencer had thousands of followers, and I had watched her content for years. That's when it hit me. I didn't notice that she wasn't wearing a bra, *so why would other people do if I stopped wearing one?*

As I didn't need support, I initially stopped wearing bras because they were more uncomfortable than anything else. Later, as I received more and more comments, I realised that the choice of wearing one or not wasn't truly mine. I started hating hearing people say, 'You shouldn't wear that; it is not decent' or 'You're not supposed to display this,' because these comments were consistently aimed at women. Gradually, challenging decency norms became one of the reasons why I didn't want to wear bras anymore. I am not implying that by wearing one, you are not fighting patriarchy; this was just my way of unlearning decency norms: by confronting them. When I decided to stop wearing it, I lived in a relatively safe suburb of Paris for a few months and my internship was in a really 'Gen Z' newsroom, so no one would judge me. Plus, it was almost winter. So, I stopped wearing bras under sweaters and long-sleeved tops where my nipples weren't too visible.

The first reaction I got was, surprisingly, from my boyfriend at the time. He came to visit me in Paris, and as we were leaving my apartment, he looked at my nipples and said, 'Why are you doing this? It's a bit provocative, don't you think?' I was perplexed to hear this coming from his mouth and asked why it would be a problem, to which he answered, 'I don't know, I just associate that with being a bit of *a tease*.' I explained to him that if heterosexual men stopped sexualising breasts, women would not need to hide them. Looking back, I did not know much about the topic then, so justifying my decision not to wear a bra was a challenging task. Plus, saying, 'It just doesn't feel right to me', did not seem a good enough reason to defy social norms. After this, I still did not wear a bra, but I felt more aware that I was going against society's rules. I remember walking and putting my arms across my chest to hide my nipples because I was not self-confident enough that day or crossing a crowded place. Sometimes I would be too self-aware and wear a cardigan to hide them again. It felt as if I was 'losing' against these rules because the pressure to conform to decency was too strong, but the truth was, I was scared. I feared people calling me an easy girl, a slut, or a tease. It felt like when you smile at someone in the street, and they come to you thinking that you are flirting, but this was simply my body existing. I feared being judged or sexually assaulted because of this. By saying no to wearing a bra, I had crossed the invisible 'decency laws' regulating French society. I was exposed and would *have asked for it* if I had been assaulted one day.

This chapter confirms that I am not the only one who has felt pressured about how I needed to dress. And, as Angela King wrote so rightly: 'Woman's crime of being other – of embodying all that man fears and despises yet desires – finds fitting "punishment" in clothing that draws erotic attention to the body by simultaneously constraining and "correcting" it.'[1]

1/ Facing the male gaze

One day, as I was walking in the street, self-conscious about my nipples being visible, I realised that no matter what clothing choices I made, they would conform to the male gaze in one way or the other. If I covered them up, I would be considered 'decent', but I would be regulated by heterosexual men's rules because they initially perceive me as a sexual object tempting them. On the other hand, if I did not cover my nipples, I would be deemed indecent and a sexual object because 'I asked for it'. Women cannot win. No matter what choice they make, they are sexualised publicly and privately until they learn to be socially invisible.

What is the male gaze?

In her essay 'Visual Pleasure and Narrative Cinema', published in 1975, Laura Mulvey, a prominent scholar and filmmaker, introduced the concept of the 'male gaze'.[2] This ground-breaking work delves into the issues of internalisation, voyeurism, and scopophilia as they affect the sexualisation and objectification of women in popular movies. In her analysis, Mulvey reveals how women are often portrayed as passive objects of sexual desire, catering to the heterosexual male viewer. These films depict women solely from the male perspective, neglecting their personal stories, thoughts, and aspirations. Instead, women's characters are reduced to superficial traits, such as the size of their breasts, disregarding their agency and individuality. Mulvey's examination of the 'male gaze' offers critical insights into how patriarchal power dynamics operate within cinema and visual media. She highlights how the objectification of women perpetuates a narrow and harmful representation that reinforces gender stereotypes and diminishes the complexity of women's experiences. Furthermore, Mulvey engages with psychoanalysis to delve deeper into the psychological implications of the 'male gaze'. She draws from concepts like voyeurism and scopophilia, which emphasise looking and deriving pleasure from looking. The male viewer's gaze becomes an active, controlling force that seeks to dominate and possess the female subject through the act of looking. This psychoanalytic perspective suggests that the 'male gaze' is rooted in deep-seated desires for power and control, which find expression through the visual representation of women as passive objects of desire.

One example of the male gaze is the creation of the *Victoria's Secret* brand. It was founded in 1977 by a man called Roy Raymond, who was frustrated with not being able to find sexier lingerie for his wife than 'floral printed nightgowns'.[3] He wanted a boudoir space with lingerie that appealed to husbands and boyfriends based on male beauty standards. However, because the focus was only on male desires, the company was almost bankrupt until it shifted to marketing the brand as a symbol of women's empowerment.[4]

But the male gaze is not limited to imposing sexy lingerie on women. It is everywhere. It is present when women try on jeans and assess whether they have a 'good enough' bottom, when women are terrified to age because their naturally wrinkled faces will be considered unattractive. It also exists when women feel the need to cover their breasts to avoid being labelled a 'slut'. Foucault described the subtle power of the male gaze on women: 'There is no need for arms, physical violence, or material constraints. Just a gaze. An inspecting gaze.'[5] This gaze becomes internalised to the point where everyone becomes controlled and controlling of others' adherence to social norms. Women feel pressure to follow the rules, becoming so aware of their breasts that they end up covering them as if they were too much. The male gaze appears to be directly linked to internalised decency since it fuels objectification and self-objectification of women. Women might perceive themselves as sexual objects without even realising it due to the way they are portrayed in advertisements, movies, music videos, and other media.[6] They may then end up internalising decency norms.

Pressure and body perception

Now that we have seen how men have sexualised breasts and bras have been used to oppress women, how does it work? How do women end up *unable to go out without wearing one?*

Women face an inspecting gaze that rules how they dress daily. Being objectified makes them feel like they need to avoid being considered indecent or even slutty, and bras play a part in making them feel like this. Since this underwear has been around for centuries through corsets, brassieres, and, more recently, push-ups, it has been eroticised and considered an essential item for girls who want to become women. Buying the first bra is regarded as a 'ritual' towards womanhood.[7] Emma, one of my interviewees aged 30, describes how bras make her think of femininity:

> In movies, it always comes down to the woman taking off her bra, and that's it. It's ideal. It's beauty. It never happens in a film that a woman takes off her panties before her bra. As if that was what you had to show first to prove your femininity.[8]

Therefore, she loves to shop for lingerie when she feels like it. It makes her feel like she owns her body and chooses how she dresses it. Like her, Tara, aged 23, explains that it makes her feel more feminine. However, she still questions why: 'Personally, it makes me feel like a woman when I have nice underwear, and I think I'm sexy. Although, what is feeling feminine apart from fulfilling social norms?'[9] In her study, Rachel Wood answers how lingerie can make women feel like they are experiencing 'real womanhood'. According to her, women 'gain pleasure from visually performing femininity as a form of love and care for a partner, to feel sexually "wanted", to enhance feelings of confidence'.[10] In addition, they feel attractive and validated by society because they perform their gender. Clara, aged 41, from a different generation than Emma, defends why push-up bras are essential for certain women to feel like they are 'women enough'. 'When you have big breasts, you don't like to show it too much, but when you have small breasts, you can be insecure because you don't feel like a real woman,' she explains.[11] However, this concept of 'being a real woman' depending on breast size might have been inherited from objectification, decency norms, capitalism, and the clever marketing strategies created to sell more and more underwear. Precisely, shaming women for having too large or tiny breasts pushes them to find a solution to the problem capitalism created so they can be sexy or decent enough.

Nevertheless, this notion of 'owning their bodies' stops where decency rules start. Emma believes bras give her confidence and help her fit French society's beauty standards. But yet, she still feels stuck:

> I felt it was an obligation. Afterwards, I took it more as a sign of femininity. That's how I show my breasts off, and I think lingerie is super pretty. The only thing I no longer impose on myself is padded bras. I'm putting on more and more bras without padding, just leaving my breasts as they are, but I still feel the need to cover them.[12]

When I asked Emma if she thinks bras oppress women, she replied, 'I would say that technically that's what it does when I come home and take it off because it hurts me, but it is a way of hiding.'[13] She adds that no matter who rings the doorbell, her first instinct is always to put on a bra. 'I've been married for ten years and always turn around when I put my bra on. Sometimes I put it on really quickly when I know he will look.'[14] Emma fears being sexualised and often feels the need to dress in black, so no one can see her breast shape. When asked about displaying her nipples, she said: 'That's the worst, genuinely the worst. Nipples are highly associated with sexualisation.'[15] In reality, nipples are one of the parts of the breast considered most sexual. Pitts-Taylor writes that 'free bouncing breasts and nipples that protrude from clothing are considered somewhat a sexual provocation.'[16]

Lucie, aged 31, explains that because of the shape of her breasts, she could not go to work without a bra because it would not feel professional enough. 'It depends where I am going,'[17] she concludes. I also asked Clara how she would react if her breasts were exposed under a light T-shirt in the street. Straightaway, she answers:

> I think I would cross my arms on my chest. I would not be very comfortable because of the transparency. If there is no one in the street, maybe I would say to myself that it is not a problem, but if there is someone, I would not be comfortable if this person saw them. I think bras camouflage breasts. It erases the pointed nipples and the pendulum movements.[18]

Noa, aged 19, does not wear bras most of the time and explains how she perceives society's obsession with hiding nipples. 'No matter the breast size, if the nipples are visible, people will start saying that *your whole breast* is visible, and it will be perceived negatively,' she explains.[19] This comment perfectly illustrates how nipples are regulated by internalised decency. Because nipples are often seen as the main sign of a natural breast showing, women are expected to wear a bra to have a smooth shape.[20]

2/ Private vs public: Belonging to heterosexual men

'Social disappearance has become, for many women in the West, the default mode of experiencing the body,' wrote Heyes.[21] The private versus public dichotomy has been a reality in Western women's lives for centuries. In 1968, women fought against this system with slogans like 'personal is political'.[22] If, for now, you do not fully understand what I am talking about, think about the people around you. Have you ever heard someone from your family or friends say, 'This girl had a *huge* cleavage at the party – her boyfriend was so mad because other guys were looking at her'? Unfortunately, many of my girlfriends have been in this situation where men made them feel guilty for displaying *their* bodies. In the mind of their – thankfully – ex-partners, women's bodies belonged to them if they were in a relationship, meaning that other people should not be able to see the same body parts they do. This is a simple example of the private versus public problem: asking women to cover their bodies publicly but pressuring them to uncover it for their partners in private.

What men gain from hiding women's bodies

Heterosexual men continue to objectify women living in Western developed countries like France and the United Kingdom. Objectification means reducing someone to an object; in this case, women are often perceived as sexual objects or fantasies. However, objectification has numerous consequences on women's lives, including participating in their oppression. I have explained how women used to be physically and mentally oppressed, reducing their chances of being anything more than wives or daughters. However, being objectified is a more subtle yet powerful form of oppression. In her article, Diane Ponterotto explains how the beauty standards created by the objectification of women also reduce their potential in life: it allows men to sexualise women and consequently not share the power they have.[23] As women are 'homogenised' and 'normalised', they are not considered individuals, and they already know how they should behave, dress, talk, or act. Because they internalise that they should see themselves as objects, it reduces the possibilities for women to access knowledge, produce knowledge or even define who they truly are. In other words, it 'denies female agency'.[24] Michel Foucault also talks about a 'race for domination', which repeats itself in history through rituals 'that impose rights and obligations', establishing a power dynamic over everything, even bodies.[25]

The irony is that women end up helping their oppressors to regulate them by doing it themselves. As they grow up, women realise they must conform to the invisible rules of femininity through their posture, behaviour, or clothes. As explained by Ponterotto in this extract:

> Men peer at women; they scrutinise and judge them; they reduce female subjectivity to a material form and expect that form to be eternally youthful, sexually attractive, physically and psychologically compliable to socially-constructed patterns of bodily form and behaviour. What enormous power lies in the objectifying consequences of this male gaze, a disciplinary gaze, which subjects and victimises women.[26]

Suppose women do not want to follow the 'rules' established and, for example, refuse to wear sexy lingerie or makeup. In that case, they 'risk failure in both the public and the private sphere, like not being successful in their workplace or not being perceived as sexual or "fulfilling" with their partners'.[27] To prove the impact of objectification on women, Fredrickson and Roberts developed the objectification theory. In two of their studies, women were more likely to treat themselves as sexual objects when they were led to believe that they would interact with a male stranger.[28] This phenomenon means that women learn to degrade themselves if they are in contact with heterosexual men to 'fit the norm'. Even in a supposed progressive and free French modern society, women's appearances are still judged and supervised because of centuries of objectification of their bodies.[29]

Because they learned decency norms, women make their breasts invisible to the point where they would be considered 'decent' but simultaneously make their entire selves disappear. As Luna Dolezal highlights in her research, this quest for physical invisibility stems from the desire to have an unobtrusive body that will pass unnoticed.[30] However, any disruption of this physical invisibility is considered pathological and necessary to eradicate. Paradoxically, despite their efforts to make their bodies invisible, women are in a state of 'permanent visibility' where they are continuously watched and judged.[31] They are told they can only wear clothing that appeals to men, and that too in private if they want to be seen as decent. By oppressing them, heterosexual men rest assured that they will not have to share their power. They subordinate women to a rank of sexual objects existing mainly for their pleasure.

Where heteronormativity meets purity culture: Your breasts are my property

I know what you are probably wondering right now. *What's this 'heteronormativity' thing?* It is when heterosexual relationships are seen as the norm, therefore putting pressure on people to engage in that type of relationship to be considered 'normal'. When heteronormativity is combined with purity culture, it creates the expectation that women should sexually please their male partner as their primary goal in life.[32] For example, women may feel pressure to buy flattering lingerie that uplifts their breasts or wear a thong, even if it can be the most uncomfortable – frankly agonising – item of clothing created. Yet, because young women internalised men's perception of them, they know what to wear to 'look attractive' and be considered sexy according to their gaze.[33] One of my interviewees, Clara, explains how she chooses her clothes because her boyfriend does not want her to be stared at by other men: 'My boyfriend is jealous, so

I dress differently; but on the other hand, he also likes me to dress sexy, so I don't know.'[34] This explanation encapsulates the 'private versus public' implicit rule that women must face. In France, flashy or 'loud' colours like red are considered highly sexual, sometimes too sexual to wear in public.[35] They are, however, socially allowed, and women are even encouraged to wear them in private for their partners. Doing so is associated with 'belonging' to only one man and is mostly seen as standard.[36] When I asked Clara how she feels about women wearing 'sexy' clothing to go out and not only for their partners, she confirmed this theory: 'Generally, women who display a big cleavage or wear sexy clothes are often single.'[37]

As Clara's sentence recounts, women are expected not to be 'too sexy' outside their relationship. They must be attractive according to the conventional rules of 'performing Western femininity' but find the right balance. This way, heterosexual men can brag about how pretty their girlfriends are without feeling threatened to 'lose her to other men' – because women are trophies, evidently. The answer seems obvious, but still: *why are women shamed for being 'too sexy'*? Because their bodies are perceived as 'territory' through the male gaze. It is, as described by Ponterotto, 'a valuable resource to be acquired' by heterosexual men.[38] Therefore, because men are conditioned to believe that women's bodies belong to them, they feel they also have the right to regulate them. An excellent example of this ownership is from a French thread on JeuxVideo.com. Several men discuss whether their girlfriends should be allowed to post pictures of their bodies on social media. The creator of this thread explains that 'his girlfriend is looking too appealing on Instagram'. Even though he 'does not want to control her', he does not like when other men can see her curves, including her breasts. One of the men answers, 'She is showing her attributes to attract as many men as possible. I hope that you are aware of that.'[39] Another thread on the same website starts with this post:

> My girlfriend started fitness six months ago, and guess what? She already wants to be a slut on Instagram. I am saying no (…), but she told me she would create one if she wanted. Am I right in saying no? If a girl is happy in her relationship, why would she show some pictures of her body on the internet? What is she going to get if strangers see her body?

The responses to this post vary from 'You should tell her what you think of the kind of women who post things like that and how you will be perceived as her boyfriend if she does' to 'Set her an ultimatum. It's not about allowing her to go out with her friends past 9 p.m.; she is literally talking about creating an Instagram account and showing her curves to horny men' or 'She can show whatever she wants, as long as it is not inappropriate in any way.'[40] In each of these comments, heterosexual men assume that women exist solely for their visual pleasure and want to be watched by men. They all ponder how disrespectful and damaging it would be for their reputations as men meant to 'own' their girlfriends if those posted their bodies on social media. Yet, they do not question if the problem might be their gaze objectifying women or consider that women can simply display their bodies as part of their *own* identity and choices.

3/ Hello capitalism

French women, on average, spend 131€ per year (£110) on lingerie,[41] with bras representing 50% of the global underwear industry sales.[42] For centuries, underwear brands have encouraged women to consume more and more, shaping social norms in the process. Lingerie marketing strategies reinforce the idea that breasts are indecent, whether because of beauty standards or because women must buy lingerie to please their partners in private settings. The commodity culture, which creates a need for anything brands want to sell, has led young girls to wear bikini tops at the beach, even before their breasts fully develop.[43] But do you know all the strategies companies use to make women feel like they should be 'decently dressed'?

I was born to seduce you

In the popular Netflix show *Emily in Paris*, Emily works for a marketing agency that decides to create a perfume advertisement. The brand's CEO,

Antoine, explains to her that the woman in the ad will walk naked on a bridge while numerous men watch her on each side. He describes this as the woman dreaming of her biggest fantasy: being sexually desired by men. After hearing the plot, Emily answers,[44] shocked:

EMILY   I didn't, uh, expect her to be naked.
CEO   She's not naked. She's wearing the perfume. It's very sexy, isn't it?
EMILY   Sexy or sexist?
CEO   I don't understand. How is this sexist?
EMILY   Well, whose dream is it anyway? The men or the woman?
CEO   It's her dream, of course. To be admired and desired by men.
EMILY   But it's the male gaze.
        (...)
CEO   What is wrong with the male gaze?
EMILY   The men are objectifying her. They have the power.
CEO   No, she has the power. Because she's beautiful and she's naked, which gives her more power.
EMILY   Maybe in her dream, she's wearing clothes.

This scene perfectly illustrates two specific aspects of marketing. First, it assumes that the primary goal of women's bodies is to be a source of sexual desire for men. Second, brands create a fake feeling of empowerment by describing a 'powerful woman' as someone men desire. Moreover, brands still imply that women are temptresses – returning to Eve in Christianity. Furthermore, campaigns that sexualise women's breasts reinforce the idea that they should be hidden: they are *so* enticing to heterosexual men that they can *even* grab their attention in an ad. An ad illustrating this concept was created and released by Nikon in France in 2009. The picture shows two women standing with different camera quality written below them. The woman on the left is shown to have smaller breasts associated with 'poor' camera quality. Meaning: the new camera is better than the previous one, and so are bigger breasts compared to smaller ones. Additionally, in this ad, her breasts have that 'nice and round shape', and her nipples are invisible to follow decency rules.

Some brands, like *Aubade*, a French female lingerie company, took the sexualisation of women to another level. They mixed the idea of 'women being perceived as sexual objects' with 'women should be sexual for their partners only' in their yearly calendars for twenty-five years. Since 1992, the brand has been giving women 'seduction tips', 183 lessons on how to keep their partners attracted to them. In numerous lessons, *Aubade* talks about 'reminding him of how fragile you are' or, like in the picture above, 'acting all innocent', written next to a woman wearing a bra. While many are widely considered sexist,[45] these displays enforce two ideas that pressure women. The first one is that they are, again, temptresses, and because they display their breasts, they are guilty of turning the man on and should not 'act all innocent'. Second, they should look sexually attractive to turn their partners on. My interviewee Carla explains how uncomfortable this kind of ad made her feel:

> There are things you don't buy to put on. The Basque, for example, is definitely worn to please men because it is not comfortable at all. When we look at old advertisements, like the lessons of *Aubade*, which spoke of attracting man's gaze, they made you understand that you had to buy lingerie to please.[46]

Emma explains how her Christian mum also made her feel like this as a teenager. 'She always explained sexuality to me brutally and falsely, saying, 'Oh, you know, you're just there to satisfy the sexual desires of men, even if you don't want to.'[47] Once she got a boyfriend, Emma bought lingerie to feel 'wanted' by him, but she quickly stopped. 'In my head, if I wanted to please my boyfriend, I had to conform to what he liked, but it felt like my body did not belong to me; it had only become the desire of others.'[48] Noa noticed that her friends also tended to buy different underwear depending on their boyfriends' choices,

> Sometimes when I speak with my friends, I hear them say it's good when there is a sexy side to lingerie. For example, one of my friends buys more and more lingerie because her boyfriend likes it. The last time we talked about it, she told me it didn't necessarily make her happy to do it.[49]

What Noa describes perfectly illustrates women's feeling that they must seduce their male partners and fit the male gaze's beauty standards.

If they do not fit the standards, they are even less decent

Heterosexual men's 'ownership' of women also includes setting beauty standards for breasts: round, high, invisible nipples, and big enough, but not too big.[50] Lucie adds, 'If it's not something men want to see, it won't be something to display.'[51] These standards generate profits for men by making women feel bad about their bodies, creating a problem that brands can solve. This has been a marketing strategy for centuries, as seen with the release of 'posture-correcting' corsets when sales of traditional corsets decreased.[52] In 1969, lingerie brands like *Exquisite Form* still employed this marketing strategy. In their advertisement, the brand wrote: 'How many times have you seen a bra or girdle that looked terrific on a model but not so terrific on you? That's because you're a woman, and a model is a mannequin,' followed by an explanation of how women could solve this problem by buying bras.[53] By writing 'every figure isn't perfect,' *Exquisite Form* and other brands promote the idea that women should strive for perfection and hide any features that do not fit contemporary Western beauty norms – including their natural breast shape. Therefore, women are pressured to wear a bra to conceal their potentially noticeable nipples, sagging breasts, and other 'imperfections' that are not considered visually acceptable. Emma, for example, hates her breasts because they are too large and go against these norms. When I ask her how she feels about push-up bras, she explains:

> These are the bras I feel the best in, even if I must put them back in place all day. But ultimately, it is the one who gives the round shape and lifts them up. When I want to show my cleavage, for example, which I don't do very often, but if I want to, the shape must be presentable, so I'm going to put on a push-up. I tried to buy basic bras, but I can't change the fact that I would always feel sexier in a push-up because that looks ideal.[54]

During the pandemic, many French women stopped wearing bras, and some have decided not to wear them again. Approximately 8% of French women were not wearing one before lockdowns, against 18% now.[55] However, the media has pressured them to think about potential sagging breasts and cleavage before ditching bras.[56] After all, what could be *worse* than seeing some sagging breasts or *actual* visible nipples on a woman? In 2016, the underwear brand *Dim* released its new bra for teenagers in France. On the tag was advertised: 'Ideal as a first bra. Hide imperfections and give a smooth breast shape.[57]' The brand was accused of conditioning young teenagers to think that showing nipples is indecent and an 'imperfection'. Noa, who does not usually wear a bra, feels like she should sometimes: 'If my breasts are sagging a bit too much or if my cleavage is too wide, I tend to wear one to push them up a little bit.'[58] However, she is aware that advertisements create insecurities and make her feel like she needs to 'correct' her appearance: 'Adverts act as if you were to wear this bra, all your insecurities would disappear,'[59] – insecurities that they, yet, themselves created.

A well-known source of entertainment aimed at French women, which uses their insecurities to generate an audience, is makeover shows. These are about performing conventional femininity and giving women the approval they deserve for fitting the norm. Makeover shows make women understand that they should hide their natural breast shape, among many other rules they are urged to follow.[60] These shows claim to be about women's power and how their insecurities should not define them. Therefore, they usually focus on the body parts these women hate to find a solution and 'fix them' – or, in other words, make them socially accepted. At the beginning of these shows, the women usually face people's judgement of them in the street. 'She's not classy or feminine' or 'She looks neglected' are the typical sentences candidates hear when going through the process. The goal? Making them understand that not performing conventional femininity is a shame, so they 'realise their mistake' and come back on the beautiful path of societal norms. After the makeover is complete, candidates usually appear in front of their partners and family wearing heels, displaying their cleavage, and conforming to every female Western beauty standard. They then listen as their peers praise how feminine and attractive they look now. By watching these shows, women might internalise that they must be 'sexy but not too sexy' to fit society's requirements. Young girls might also internalise decency norms by watching women with ample cleavage or revealing clothes described as 'not classy' or 'too much' and women wearing a tracksuit as 'neglected' or 'unattractive'.

As a whole, brands make women feel bad about their bodies to sell more products and convince them they would be more confident if they 'corrected' their breasts. Unfortunately, modern Western society does not encourage women to accept their bodies to feel empowered. Instead, empowerment is associated with wearing a bra that conforms to societal norms, while women are led to believe they are in control since they can choose the patterns on their underwear.

Fake empowerment is the new cash cow

The notion of empowerment is not only used to sell bras that correct women's insecurities about their bodies. Recently, empowerment has been associated with 'norms-free women' in advertisements. However, the women in these ads are not free to wear a bra only if they want to. They just wear the type of lingerie usually perceived as 'provocative' but, this time, to 'please themselves'.[61] Clara, one of my participants, commented that it is a way to 'express who we are' when asked how she feels about lingerie ads advocating for 'empowerment'.[62] However, this trend mostly happened because of increased awareness about capitalism and the male gaze. Like manufacturers did when corset sales decreased, brands adapted to feminism to avoid losing the market.

A perfect example is the contested *Wonderbra*'s 'Hello boys' ad, which was turned in 2018 into 'Hello me'. French women denounced the 'new sexism' happening here, adding that the problem would not be solved by still pressuring women to be sexy and hiding it behind a new slogan.[63] Lucie explains that 'it spreads the idea that we must buy something to love our bodies. They noticed that society wasn't accepting sexism anymore, so they had to find something else.'[64] This new way to promote goods and products is called 'ad-her-tising'. It is described as 'female-targeted advertising that exhibits qualities of empowering women, female activism or women leadership'.[65] Researcher Alyssa Baxter explains in her research article that ad-her-tising is much more than brands encouraging women to buy more. They are also 'taking advantage of feminism as a legitimate source of activism. The goal of the companies is to make the consumer believe they are passionate about a cause while not necessarily believing in the messages they publicise.'[66] As proof, her study develops two fair points. First, the feminist stance of the brand is contradicted by the products they sell. This statement applies to the *Wonderbra* ad 'Hello me', apparently destined to symbolise women's empowerment. However, the brand sells lingerie designed according to the male gaze beauty criteria and still calls its bras a 'solution' for women.[67] The second point made by the study is that the male-targeted ads created by the same brands that tried to empower women are male-centred again:

> Women in the male-targeted advertisements analysed said no more than one sentence in each ad. The women were also either scantily clad in bikinis, presented as a prize in a tight-fitting evening dress, or shown in what is commonly discussed as one of a man's favourite outfits, a sundress. The images of women in these advertisements show the opposite of feminist ideals and contradict their sister company's efforts to promote female empowerment.

Women have been sexualised in ads for centuries by heterosexual men who assume they were born to entice them. These men capitalise on either the insecurities they have generated by objectifying women or on a fake notion of empowerment that still fulfils their gaze. In both cases, the pressure on women to please men does not change. Jill Fields explains that the dominant group – here, heterosexual men – impose general directions on social life and enjoy this prestige because of their position in the world of production. As men mainly direct the Western market, they get all the benefits while oppressing women.[68]

Conclusion

Almost all the women interviewed felt that wearing a bra was a burden they used mainly to hide their insecurities or avoid being criticised for having visible nipples. The need to hide comes from the pressure men create to have power over women and reduce their chances of thinking of themselves as something other than objects. Although Christianity has been decreasing in France in the twenty-first century, women are still implicitly expected to 'belong' to the man they are in a relationship with and not display their breasts, among other body parts, to other men. Norms are made clear on the internet and even in women's minds as they have been repeated throughout their lives. However, while women are pressured to dress 'decently enough', they are also expected to wear sexy lingerie to enhance certain features and be attractive. They must hide some aspects of their bodies while still highlighting others to be accepted by society. For example, they are encouraged to correct their sagging breasts if they are deemed not 'good enough' to be displayed. If they do not, they may be considered morally and aesthetically indecent. You got it by now; capitalism makes women feel like their breasts should be hidden but still attractive because, unsurprisingly, all the benefits return to … *men*.

CHAPTER 3

Social media and objectification of women's breasts

> From the moment they begin to show, a female discovers
> that her breasts are claimed by others.
>
> – Millsted and Frith[1]

One day, I was wandering in the city centre of Marseille with a friend. It was busy, and as it was after the first Covid lockdown in 2020, I had not worn a bra in months, despite the summer season. I completely forgot that I wasn't wearing one, the feeling of wearing it, or even the simple thought that my nipples could show easily. But people didn't forget. They didn't forget that not wearing a bra was a social sin and that, mainly because my summer clothes were tight, my nipples were too visible. But what was different from all the other times? As my friend and I walked down that street, I was suddenly brought back to reality by a group of men approaching me. They looked at me sexually and acted like they were coming to talk to me. I started freaking out and managed to avoid them, but my friend got a bit scared for me and asked, 'Are you comfortable walking through places like this without a bra?' Before adding, 'I am not saying that you shouldn't, but are you able to identify where or when it is safe and where or when it is not?'

From that moment on, I kept asking myself: *Where was my limit*? How far would I be willing to go 'just' to feel comfortable with my clothing choices? I eventually got my answer when heading to a restaurant in Porto, Portugal. A group of men trying to sell drugs to tourists surrounded me, but I politely declined and escaped through the crowd. I walked a bit faster as they were a large group and we were in one of the city's busiest streets. As I looked back at one of them to say no, he grabbed his genitals and stared directly into my eyes while licking his lips in a grossly aroused way. I was petrified because of a man for the first time. I knew that if I walked back home alone one day and bumped into him, what I saw in this man's eyes was everything I would be terrified of: his misogyny and the confidence that he could do anything he wanted without caring about the person in front of him. In a few seconds, I had been sexualised and objectified. For a few days after this experience, I wondered if I should have been dressed differently or worn a bra. Until I reached this conclusion: if I were to get sexually assaulted, no bra or other underwear would save me. Being braless is not the only thing that could make a man think I am trying to tease him with my appearance. I could be wearing a blouse or even some joggers, but misogynistic men like him would still have no respect for women.

I also spent a lot of time wondering what I considered 'too much' for social media, as being indecent was one of my main fears for a while. Once, I posted a picture where my cleavage was visible, and it was clear that I was naked. I loved the artistic side of this picture; the light and the composition were so beautiful. It took me so much time to ponder if I would post it until the question, 'Do I want to be that kind of girl?' came to my mind. So, I posted it simply to fight this idea. I would be 'that type of girl' and post what I wanted with my body. And if someone had asked me why I posted a picture where my breasts were visible, I would question them on who decided what body part was okay to display. Later, I uploaded a video on Tiktok where I was dancing with my friend. As I wasn't wearing a bra, the bottom part of my breast became briefly visible as we spun. My nipple wasn't visible, nor was my entire breast, only a bit of flesh. A few days later, my video got taken down for 'nudity and sexual activity'. It made me realise, once again, that choosing whether to display my own body was not entirely my decision. And this time, it wasn't my mum or friends telling me off; it was one of the world's most popular social media platforms.

Being a woman means being intensely visible. It is a paradox: women must make their bodies disappear while still seeing them being over-exposed in culture and media.[2] This contradiction is particularly evident when it comes to posting online. Women must try to be 'attractive and free' but not too much; otherwise, they would be judged or insulted. When discussing social media, it is difficult to forget the main issues affecting women: censorship, slut-shaming and cyber-harassment. By failing to monitor or openly support these issues, social media platforms send a clear message to women: 'You should internalise decency norms.'

1/ Should I post it?

I have pondered this question thousands of times. Social media reflects offline internalised decency norms regarding women's breasts. However, not everyone agrees on what is considered 'too sexy' to be worn or posted.

Hypersexualisation and female empowerment

Social media was created at the beginning of the twenty-first century,[3] bringing with it a new playground where humans can interact. Before social media, women were commonly sexualised, particularly throughout the twentieth century and mainly after the Second World War, when their breasts became objects of visual pleasure. Fashion, aesthetics, and television outlets established a sexual canon represented by women, using the sexualised female figure to promote and sell different products.[4] Consequently, some women felt pressured to dress in a way that satisfied the male gaze. As researchers argue, most women in the music industry, pornography, or reality TV have been trying to conform to these 'hypersexualised models of femininity' portrayed in the media.[5] For instance, Nicki Minaj's music video called 'Anaconda' has been heavily criticised because of all the sexual references and the male gaze point of view that the singer chose.[6] This music video summarises how heterosexual men usually portray women – in the kitchen wearing a 'sexual' outfit, with footage focusing on bottoms and breasts moulded in push-up bras. As Nicki Minaj herself explains, she 'sells sex appeal'.[7] However, researchers worry that creating more content like this could lead to the hypersexualisation of young women, pressuring them into self-objectifying.[8] Some pictures on social media are now described as 'porn chic' and sometimes involve underage girls. This phenomenon, called 'hypersexualisation', is defined as 'girls being depicted or treated as sexual objects and sexuality that is inappropriately imposed on girls through media, marketing or products directed at them that encourages them to act in adult sexual ways'.[9] Because Western society objectifies women's bodies in the media, movies, and many other platforms, girls might learn to self-objectify from a young age. This is what Fredrickson & Roberts describe in their objectification theory. 'Sexual objectification experiences are thought to socialise girls and women to treat themselves as objects to be looked upon and evaluated based upon bodily appearance. This internalisation of an observer's perspective upon one's own body is called self-objectification.'[10] By monitoring their appearance to fit beauty standards, young girls might learn to consider themselves objects and get their self-worth from male validation. Since they watched their icons being rewarded for their physical attributes, it became more common for girls to recreate identical posts with their own bodies on Instagram.[11] Thus, they might have internalised that they should self-objectify as their favourite artists do.

An article by Sonia Suarez also argues that female empowerment might have been used against women on social media.[12] For example, she wonders if women might subconsciously post their bodies on Instagram because of the male gaze, even though they justify it as them 'owning their bodies':

> This 'progressive' idea of empowerment allows us to break away from all these conservative rules, continuing to replicate them now with 'freedom', with 'our consent', and with a lot of men 'allied' who continue to look at us again as an object, without changing anything. Many types of industries, such as porn, music, film, and video games, have reinforced and created an ideal of a woman that we should all aspire to, an ideal that is moulded 100% to male comfort and pleasure and this ideal is sold to us so that we women feel even empowered to achieve it.

This article implicitly raises one question: *are women going towards a modern way of belonging to heterosexual men while thinking they are breaking free?* Daniels and Zurbriggen argue that if society equates 'subjective enjoyment' with empowerment, it neglects 'the oppressive cultural, economic, and political factors that govern women's bodies'.[13]

However, while this theory explores why women may post such content on social media, it should not lead to the conclusion that it is women's responsibility to resist the male gaze by not posting content men could 'enjoy'. Women are free to dress as they please, and it is men's responsibility to stop objectifying them. Additionally, what is deemed sexy or hypersexualised is not universal and varies from country to country and even from person to person. Thus, what might be seen as 'appealing to the male gaze' in Suarez's article could be wearing a push-up bra for one person or displaying a natural breast shape for another.

What is 'too much' according to the French?

Each country, region, and person has a different idea of what they consider 'too much'. When interviewing the women participating in this study, I noticed a spectrum of what is considered sexual, going hand in hand with what they consider decent or not. The first point of view I heard was that women wearing push-up bras or any other clothing item commonly 'required' to fit the male gaze is linked to hypersexualisation. Andréa, aged 55, does not wear a bra and insists on how covering underage girls' breasts was indecent to her:

> I follow some influencers, and I'm horrified by what I see. They hypersexualise their children by making them wear bikini tops and bras when their breasts have just started to develop, and they don't even realise it. Whether it's about bras or anything else, the problem is that all the options were created to either hide women or show them off. And these children find themselves hypersexualised by their parents, posing in a way men would like. Women who dress in a manner considered 'sexy', is that real freedom, or is it submission?[14]

Éléana, aged 18, and a completely different generation to Andréa, also shares the same opinion: 'Someone who wears a push-up at eight years old for me is hypersexualisation, but someone of any age who posts a picture without a bra, I do not consider that too sexual. Hypersexualisation for me comes from adults.'[15] On the other side of the argument, I encountered women who believe that displaying the natural shape of breasts without covering them up or making them too visible is what indecency is about. According to them, it can create the impression that they are trying to look attractive to men. Tara, 23, explains her views:

> It bothers me when I see the person trying to make their breasts stand out because it gives the impression that there is only that to see in a woman. There's a difference between a person who's going to put on something super tight without a bra with ample cleavage and a girl who just doesn't wear a bra because she doesn't care. I think we see the difference. I get the impression that the first ones feel that they know what they must display to lure men.[16]

Tara's explanation highlights a 'noticeable' difference between an 'indecent' outfit and a 'normal' one based on why women choose to wear them. It shows how both sides agree on one thing – they all reject anything that overtly signals, 'I am trying to appeal to men' – regardless of the specific item of clothing they consider to be responsible for this. Yet, these women blame totally different factors. The first group only blamed hypersexualisation on the clothing items imposed by the male gaze but did not find anything indecent. In contrast, the second group blamed indecency and hypersexualisation on women's bodies. However, statistically, a higher number of women (six out of ten participants) said that indecency was linked to breasts being too visible or braless.

To establish what would be considered indecent on social media, I asked all my participants to tell me what they thought when seeing the following: a picture of a woman with cleavage, a woman in lingerie, a woman wearing some shorts and a brassiere, a woman in bikini, a woman wearing a top with her nipples visible, and an artistic nude. It quickly became apparent that the answers were the same as what they considered indecent in public, meaning that social media is not exempt from the same decency norms. The two women aged 18 to 20 who did not wear bras anymore believed nothing in this list was indecent. Still, they felt hypersexualisation came from wearing push-up bras and Western society displaying women in outfits that conventionally appeal to the male gaze. Most women aged 21 to 45 I interviewed wore a bra daily and struggled to go out without one. For them, some of these statements – like posting visible nipples through a top – could be acceptable depending on their purpose. But for one participant in particular, Tara, posting a picture in lingerie or with ample cleavage could be considered indecent. Clara and Julia added that some of these statements could be particularly indecent if posted to show off their bodies. For this age group, indecency arises when women display some parts of their breasts that they 'should socially be hiding' since it could make men think that they want attention. Julia, 38, explains, 'What I'm going to find maybe more provocative is when enticing is the purpose. Posting a picture where your nipples are visible under a top means you want to create a reaction.'[17] Finally, women aged 46 to 60 shared the same opinion as the ones aged 18 to 20 and were even more resistant, for some of them, to the sexualisation of women that makes them wear 'sexy' clothing. However, they did not find any statements from the list indecent.

There are several explanations for why the interviewees aged 18 to 20 and 46 to 60 had a different opinion from those aged 21 to 45. First, women aged 46 to 60 grew up in the years following the sexual revolution of May 1968, and some of them saw their families becoming more liberated regarding nudity. For example, Andréa, 55, recalls that she often saw her mum naked and that nudity was never taboo for her growing up. Thus, it made her internalise different decency norms than others. Second, although women aged 18 to 20 belong to a different generation than the ones aged 46 to 60, they share similar values. Like the older group that grew up after May 1968, Generation Z was raised during the Fourth feminist wave, which is currently occurring in France and other Western countries. This new wave began in 2012 and is more focused on gender norms, especially topics related to online and offline gender equality.[18] This age group may also be more attuned to women's empowerment because they grew up following the #MeToo movement, which began in 2006. As a result, many women began speaking out against behaviours or comments that were inappropriate and unacceptable.[19] The French Gen Z also experienced the French equivalent of the #MeToo movement, called #BalanceTonPorc, in 2017.[20] They grew up listening to highly influential artists like Angèle, one of the French symbols of feminism, who is especially renowned for her song *Balance ton quoi*, which discusses hidden sexism and sexual harassment.[21] Because of all the social changes these two generations went through, the decency norms they internalised may have differed from those of the other age groups studied.

Overall, what people consider hypersexualised is subjective and may be based on the decency norms they internalised based on their generation and place of upbringing. However, all the women interviewed reject anything they perceive as 'being used to attract heterosexual men', whether their definition of indecency involves hidden or displayed breasts. Some reject bras and any item commonly used to conform to male gaze standards imposed on women, such as push-up bras, while others – the majority – reject nudity because it appears attention-seeking. Despite the differences in decency norms they internalised, their answers all show that what they find indecent is anything that is made to overtly 'accommodate the male gaze'.

2/ 'Your story goes against our community guidelines'

Decency rules on social media are similar to those applied in real life. However, what happens when social media guidelines make these unofficial decency norms a reality by censoring women's breasts on their platforms? Policies like censorship, associated with a lack of regulation, can generate slut-shaming and cyber-harassment towards women.

Social media's censorship of nipples

If you are on social media, you may have noticed that platforms like Instagram, Facebook, and Tiktok censor women's nipples and breasts. This means that almost no picture can be posted where these body parts are visible without being taken down a few hours later. In 2015, Instagram allowed breasts to be visible in breastfeeding photos only in response to protests.[22] However, several problems have arisen from these 'decency guidelines' still applied to all the non-breastfeeding images. First, only women's nipples are considered indecent and worth censoring. Second,

Instagram has been criticised for not fighting as hard against racism and hateful content as it fights against women's nipples.[23] Finally, not changing the guidelines might confirm to the offline world that this body part should not be visible. The choice to focus exclusively on women's nipples has been justified by the sexual dimension breasts hold for many communities worldwide.[24] 'We are trying to reflect the sensitivities of the broad and diverse array of cultures and countries across the world in our policies,' explained Instagram's spokesperson.[25] Several criteria help the bots to detect if the nipples are male or female, and the picture is then censored if 'necessary'. However, as expected, this rule poses a problem for non-binary or transgender people with breasts.[26] Instagram responded that if the person is non-binary, their nipples would be allowed to be displayed once the picture is reviewed. However, if it is a trans woman, her nipples would be censored.

Nevertheless, by letting people like Donald Trump share their hateful thoughts on social media for years before banning them while forbidding women from displaying their nipples, social media plays a part in reinforcing decency norms. 'There are worse things on social media, but we censor nipples. And in the end, the fact that we censor them confirms to society that they are indecent and should not be shown even though men have the same,' adds Noa, 19, one of my participants.[27] Indeed, Facebook's ban on videos of extreme violence, for example, was lifted in 2013 and justified by the awareness created by these videos.[28] However, social media platforms do not consider changing their rules regarding breasts and fighting against the sexualisation and objectification of women's bodies.[29]

Slut-shaming and harassment

Censoring women's nipples on social media and in real life can easily lead to slut-shaming and harassment. Slut-shaming is defined in the book called *What You Really Really Want* as 'language and behaviours that are intended to make women and girls feel bad about being sexual'.[30] Obviously, decency rules and purity culture have had a consequential impact on the rise of slut-shaming online and offline.[31] One example of slut-shaming and harassment linked to internalised decency is people's reactions to Janet Jackson's show during the Super Bowl of 2004 when Justin Timberlake accidentally exposed her nipple. The initial plan was for Justin to display Janet's lace bra, which collapsed and revealed her breast.[32] After this event, this unplanned incident generated many comments on how indecent Janet Jackson was. Because of it, she was uninvited from the Grammy's, blacklisted from many radio or TV channels, and widely insulted on social media for having her nipples uncovered.[33] This incident perfectly illustrates how paradoxical breasts are in Western societies. They must be hidden because of norms and seen as indecent but are still over-sexualised.[34] Moreover, this hypersexualisation extends even further when examining the Black women's experiences. Historically, Black women's bodies have been subjected to an especially powerful form of sexualisation, often rooted in racist stereotypes perpetuated by colonialism and slavery.[35] These stereotypes have reinforced harmful narratives that portray Black women as inherently more sexually promiscuous or available, contributing to a culture of objectification and dehumanisation.[36] This complex dynamic becomes evident in instances where Black women, like Janet Jackson, face amplified levels of scrutiny and backlash for similar incidents. The reactions to such incidents reveal a double standard that not only polices women's bodies but also intersects with racial bias, further compounding the challenges faced by Black women.

Catherine McCormack's seminal work *Women in the Picture* acknowledges that women from both white and Black racial backgrounds have faced objectification. She critically examines an additional layer of primitivism and wanton sexuality attributed specifically to women of colour, with a particular focus on Black women.[37] French colonialism, as an example, played a pivotal role in shaping the enduring objectification of women from the Global South, including the African and Caribbean regions. Colonialists often portrayed women of colour as emblematic of 'wanton sexuality', a term that has historically been used to describe perceived excessive or uncontrolled sexual desire or behaviour.[38] With regard to women, it has often been used pejoratively to suggest moral promiscuity or lustfulness. During colonial and slavery eras, European colonial powers and slaveholders depicted women of colour, especially Black women, as possessing wanton sexuality. This portrayal was rooted in racial prejudices and aimed at justifying the exploitation of these women. Moreover, European powers often framed the cultures of colonised peoples, including the clothing and behaviours of women, as morally inferior.[39] This perspective led to the portrayal of colonised women as exotic and excessively sexual. As McCormack explains, these narratives were employed to justify the exploitation and subjugation of Black women, and they reinforced harmful stereotypes that persist to this day, whether in the media or even in popular culture. Therefore, Black women face a unique double burden due to the intertwined stereotypes of both race and gender. Not only do they struggle with the racialised notion of hypersexuality, but they also face gender-specific challenges tied to objectification and the policing of their bodies. This has had a profound impact on how women of colour, especially Black women, are perceived and treated in society, where their bodies are often unjustly labelled as overly sexualised.

Based on my participants' responses, I noticed that their main concern when posting was that people's online reactions would be more aggressive and persistent than in person. Slut-shaming and cyber-harassment often target those who show their bodies online. One participant, Éléana, explains the difference she senses between social media and reality in terms of expectations:

> I think that, on social media, we accept more easily that girls show their bodies since society wants that, but on the other hand, we are more criticised for it. So, I think the paradox is much more on social media because, in everyday life, people aren't going to share their opinions too loudly.[40]

As she details, the paradox between women having to show their bodies enough to be enticing while following decency rules is happening both in real life and online. However, researcher Jessica Ringrose explains that there is a specific way for women to post online if they want to be considered decent on social media. 'Girls must make complex "choices" about how they will construct a sexual digital identity, with contradictory worries about how to be desirable but not "too" slutty,' she explains.[41] The tensions she describes show that women and girls must reach a balance to post online and be considered 'respectable'. They must balance decency norms and what is deemed hypersexualised in their country while being pressured to post increasingly 'desirable' content to please the male gaze and not feel left out.[42] In Paris, based on my interviews, avoiding slut-shaming means that women should not display any sign of nudity or visible sexy underwear. Doing so could be seen as 'openly trying to be enticing to men'; therefore, they would be considered a 'tease'. Thus, these women internalise that breasts must be as discreet as possible while looking desirable by being high, large, and round.

One thing the women I interviewed noted when showing their bodies on Instagram is the number of people, mainly heterosexual men, sexualising them in private messages. One of my participants, Lucie, adds that it is one of the main reasons she never posts a picture of herself on these platforms: 'I think people feel freer on social media. They are already unfiltered in the street, but it's even worse online.'[43] Almost all the women I have spoken to fear being slut-shamed. In 2020, 59% of girls aged 15–25 worldwide were abused or insulted on social media, while 41% were harassed.[44] When I asked my participants if they would rather post a picture where their breasts were visible online or wear the same outfit to go into town, many of them, like Éléana, said they would fear social media even more. 'In real life, I can mentally prepare myself and know which street I choose. Anyone can screenshot my posts online; I have no idea where they could be shared. I don't want to be insulted, for example.'[45] A study found that Instagram was the social media platform that generated the highest rate of harassment and slut-shaming.[46] Twitter was also ranked among the most violent social media platforms because of its public exposition. However, sometimes slut-shaming on Instagram can be invisible and can, for example, be done through 'raids'. People add a girl to several private group chats where she would be insulted, slut-shamed, or even receive death threats.[47] For some women with a larger audience on social media, it can become dangerous offline if some people find their home addresses and send threats or insults.

3/ Scared or sacred?

Eighty-six per cent of French women were victims of street harassment in 2018.[48] This percentage is terrifying, and the lack of regulation on social media, along with decency rules, slut-shaming, purity culture, and many other social factors, create an unsafe space for women to exist.

Where objectification and violence against women meet

For a minority of the women I interviewed, posting online is still less scary than facing people's reactions and potential violence in the street. Noa, one of them, explains that the internet creates a distance that could feel like safety: 'On social media, you can put it on private, but if I wear something in the street, anyone can check me out or come and talk to me.'[49] Social media reflects the offline world regarding decency rules; however, its lack of regulation over misogynistic posts and censorship of women's bodies contributes to objectification, which, in turn, increases violence.[50] A recent example perfectly illustrates how a whole community of toxic heterosexual men can be created and oppress women without social media reacting: the Andrew Tate scandal. If you have not heard of him, Andrew Tate is a kickboxer accused of being the head of a prostitution group. He has now been banned from social media, but he spent the entire summer of 2022 sharing his thoughts on how women should belong to men or be considered sluts if they do not.[51] Among his posts, Andrew Tate talked about sexual harassment and violence against women: 'If you put yourself in a position to be raped, you must bear some responsibility. If I left a million dollars outside my front door – when it got stolen, people would say, "Why was it there? Irresponsible." '[52] This kind of post encourages rape culture but also promotes victim-blaming because of how women dress. The biggest problem with Andrew Tate is that social media allowed him to post many misogynistic contents for three months before banning him. In the meantime, his videos have been watched more than 11.6 billion times,[53] reaching 4.7 million followers on Instagram before he was banned.[54] This story also raises significant concerns about how many men agreed with what Andrew Tate was sharing, especially after he talked about how to be violent with women if they do not 'listen to him'. As Patricia Mélotte, a Belgian sociologist, explains, online and offline worlds mirror and influence each other:

> Social media reproduce the same failings as in the physical public space. It is the reproduction of what is happening offline – meaning sexist harassment, sexualised or not, intrusive behaviours that refer to gender stereotypes. It's always the same idea of 'putting women in their place', a reminder to follow gender norms and traditional roles of men and women.[55]

But the lack of regulation on essential topics like misogyny can increase the danger for women on social media. Since these platforms can quickly bring together dangerous people and indoctrinate them easily, they potentially increase offline violence against women.

'I'm scared it's too noticeable'

Due to offline and online decency rules, some women feel uncomfortable walking in the street with their breasts too noticeable. Offline sexual harassment includes various acts, from whistling, insulting, and calling out to touching a woman's body without her consent. It is essential to consider all these acts as violence against women because they remove them from public spaces. Researchers explain that 'these acts are, at the minimum, symbolic violence with significant effects. They are intertwined with the fear which forces numerous women to elaborate strategies to avoid and exclude themselves from certain places of public space during certain hours.'[56] For example, this removal from society happens to many women who feel too vulnerable or in danger to return home at night, so they choose not to go out.[57] It also removes women's freedom to dress however they want to, as they must be 'unnoticeable' to avoid danger. The researcher Carol Brooks Gardner confirms this argument in her book when she writes that 'public harassment reinforces the division between sexes and allows the presence of one while punishing the other'.[58] This punishment occurs, for instance, when French campaigns for women's safety in public spaces encourage them to dress differently to not be identifiable as a woman – meaning that they are expected to go against what modern French society expects from a 'feminine' outfit.[59] These campaigns often use phrases like 'do not be noticeable,'[60] which can lead women to internalise that in addition to following decency norms to be socially accepted, they must also follow them to stay safe, or they could be blamed for it.

When I asked my participants whether they would feel more protected against sexual assault on the street if they wore a bra, some immediately responded that it would not impact the outcome. For example, Lucie said:

> If the woman doesn't wear one, they will say that it was the reason she got assaulted, but if she did, they would say it is because the strap was visible or it was too sexy. So they will always find an excuse to make us believe that if we hide the breast's shape, we are protected when really we aren't.[61]

However, for most of them, wearing a bra feels like psychological protection, providing an extra layer to prevent a potential assaulter from accessing their breasts. Emma explains:

> I've had a lot of situations in the tube where the person is just pressed against my breasts or guys say gross things in your ear. And that's also why I'm scared. My fear of not wearing a bra in the street comes from there. I'm afraid it's more noticeable. There are still more women who wear bras than women who do not, so it is necessarily more apparent, and I don't want to be noticed, watched all the time, or judged. We always hear, 'ok, it's not a reason to rape her, but still.' The more layers, the more protected I feel. If I wear a dress, I will put on a tank top underneath to hide the cleavage to feel safe.[62]

For Romane, 51, the movement of her breasts sometimes makes her feel more vulnerable. However, she concludes the same as Éléana; it is more about being mentally reassured than anything else:
I think when it comes to street harassment, sometimes you get less hassle when you wear a bra, but I think it wouldn't make a big difference; it's more psychological, I guess. But again, it depends on the bra because

I think that, unfortunately, the more you emphasise cleavage, the more you tend to feel in danger.[63]

Women are constantly assessing whether their cleavage is too broad, whether their nipples are showing too much, or if they should hide their bodies to avoid harassment, assault, or danger. Decency norms create a climate in which women continually fear being noticed and harassed.

Conclusion

Online and offline decency rules often mirror each other. However, social media fails to control misogynistic content, contributing to increasing violence against women. Social media platforms ban nipples, but there is no regulation for people like Andrew Tate, who actively shares hate speech towards women and needs to be banned quickly. These unregulated, hateful online communities can also encourage or support violence towards women offline while reinforcing decency norms. What could be more powerful to force women to hide their bodies than to make them fear being assaulted or insulted if they don't? Women become victims of what misogynistic people like Andrew Tate share on social media: their bodies are deemed too sexual to be displayed. So, if they were to get assaulted, it would be their problem because, as Tate says, 'If he left a million dollars outside his front door – when it got stolen, people would say, "Why was it there? Irresponsible," ' *right*?

CHAPTER 4

Women vs women

I wouldn't like them to think 'What the fuck is this one doing?'
– My participant, Lucie, about other women's opinion[1]

During the summer of 2019, I had to move back in with my parents for a few months. While my mum is now one of my strongest allies, it took both her and my dad a few years to truly grasp that women might feel pressured to wear a bra, whether they need it for support or not. Eventually, they became highly supportive and educated themselves on the topic. However, in 2019, neither of them understood why I felt the need to 'go against the rules'. My mum used to tell me that it looked 'dirty' or 'indecent and neglected' before I went out. After several arguments, we agreed they would stop talking about it, which worked until my birthday. We were going to a fancy restaurant with my grandparents, and my mum opened my bedroom door, looked at me up and down and said, 'Could you just do it for today? Your clothing choices are inappropriate now because I don't like being stared at. When being with you *like that* in public, I feel like people are watching us because *this* is not the norm.' From that point, I again questioned myself a lot. If anything, she communicated her issue clearly. It was more about her wanting to be invisible than about me not wearing a bra. But why was I pressured into decency? Should I comply with the 'rules' if they make me uncomfortable so that I do not make others uncomfortable? And more particularly, did they have a good reason to be uncomfortable *because my nipples' shape was showing through my clothes*? I considered changing, but deep down, I knew that 'decency' wasn't an acceptable reason to cover myself up, nor was it equal. And I knew social norms would never change if no one ever made people uncomfortable. So, I went to that birthday meal, dressed precisely how I wanted.

Later that summer, I put on my swimsuit at the beach and realised that a part of me still felt the need to hide my breasts because I could only imagine going topless when people weren't around. I feared conflicts, especially with other women who could come up to me and ask me to dress up because it was indecent for their children to see *that*. I felt ready to stop wearing a bra only when I knew people had no right telling me what to do. But at that exact moment, I wasn't sure if someone could ask me to cover myself. While topless is officially allowed in France for women, numerous police officers have arrested, fined, or even just asked women to dress up because they found it indecent. It wasn't based on any law but purely on peer pressure. And, as much as I loved fighting the idea that my breasts were an inappropriate body part, I didn't like having to debate it with strangers. Fast forward two years later. It was 2021, and I was fully confident about not wearing a bra. Even when wearing the tightest tops or the ones quite see-through, I didn't care; I wasn't even noticing it anymore. I wasn't seeing people make funny faces when realising that I wasn't wearing one. But one fear remained: would I be allowed to dress that way in a workplace? That summer, I applied to work with a language travel exchange company and got in. As I was packing to work with them, I remember feeling so anxious that someone might make comments about my clothing choices. I pondered packing some for ages. *What if I got fired*? After a thorough search on Google, I calmed down and realised that, realistically, no one could fire me because I wasn't wearing a bra. But as I closed my suitcase, I slid two bras to the side. The pressure won. I wasn't ready to dress the way I wanted and expose my 'indecent breasts'.

In both scenarios, peer pressure made me doubt myself and feel like I did not fit the norm. All the women I interviewed also expressed a fear of judgement and self-doubt, stemming from people's opinions on the street, in school, and even within their own families. Women have internalised the misogyny around them to the point where they now judge and pressure each other to conform to decency norms that oppress them all. Girls are expected not to display their bras and to choose the right colours to avoid appearing 'immoral'. And more often than not, their families are the first environment to sexualise them without their consent.

1/ Mirror, mirror on the wall, who is the sexiest of them all?

Women are often socially divided into two categories: the respectable and the slut, with their clothes defining which category they belong to. While some women would like to believe that slut-shaming is only initiated by heterosexual men and that women only support each other, the reality is that women can also be quick to criticise their girlfriends. Who has never heard a group of girls talking about one another and saying, 'Her skirt is so short today; she's really craving attention' or 'She is having sex with too many people to respect herself.' These comments are a product of internalised misogyny and slowly bully women into following decency norms.

What kind of woman do you want to be?

As one of my participants, Noa, recounts, it is a 'well-known social rule' in France that women should not have their breasts visible in public, or they will hear 'some comments like "Oh, your nipples are showing," and "be careful, your breast is visible," which make you understand that you have to be careful because people could look at you'.[2] This pressure is associated with having a good reputation in some Western countries like France, where sexual attractiveness has become a means of rating women to know if they will be socially accepted. Therefore, only the women who adhere to social norms will be seen as deserving of the success associated with women: getting married, having a family, and giving birth.[3]

Nevertheless, responding to the norm correctly is also essential. Sexual attractiveness depends on each person's perception and is regulated by different decency norms from one country to another, making it even harder to fit standards. For the French women I interviewed, the fear of being judged, even if it is a simple look, makes them regulate how they dress in an even stricter way. For example, when I gave Tara a scenario where she would be walking down the street wearing Jeans and a light t-shirt without a bra and asked her what her thoughts would be at that exact moment, she answered:

T   I would think 'dress up' and tell myself everyone is looking at it, and they all
    think I want to show off my breasts.
R   Why is it wrong to want to show them off?
T   It gives off this image of the girl trying to get attention.[4]

Unfortunately, Tara could be right. According to a poll conducted in
France, 39% of French men surveyed think that a woman not wearing a
bra is trying to attract their gaze.[5]

But where does the problem come from? As mentioned, purity culture and heteronormativity can make women feel they should only show
their bodies to their heterosexual male partners. It also stigmatises women
for being sexually active, especially if it is not with a 'stable partner'. This
stigma extends to clothes that are considered symbols of 'sexual availability'.[6]
The result is slut-shaming, where women are openly shamed for wearing
specific clothes or acting in a particular way. For example, a study found
that dressing in a 'provocative' way – with nipples visible, for instance –
is perceived as a symbol of sexual availability.[7] Thus, if the person being
slut-shamed was dressed in that way, the slut-shamer would be judged less
harshly for being mean because their opinion would be seen as warranted.
My participant, Andréa, mentioned what is called in French the 'Madone
versus putain' dichotomy. As she explains, 'For certain people, it is still
about the story of the mother and the slut; we must be one or the other
but not both. But it is wrong. We are both.'[8] In French, the word 'putain'
represents an immoral woman who is sexually active with several partners
and not worth being respected, which is what displaying breasts and nipples is often associated with.[9] On the other hand, the 'mother' represents
a respectable woman.[10] As a study on slut-shaming explains:

> We see appearing a polarisation between women: the good ones who are the ones
> that need to be defended, and the bad ones, the others. There are also two figures: the
> girl that guys hang out with and can introduce as their partner and the one they
> occasionally see to have sex. It shows the dichotomy between two types of women
> who are seen in society as having two different roles and, especially, an opposite le-
> gitimacy from each other.[11]

This opposition is omnipresent in how French women's clothes are assessed. As my participant Emma explains, it is about judgement, no matter what women wear. 'If I display my cleavage, I would be considered a slut. If I'm wearing too many layers, I am prudish.'[12]

When decency becomes a competition

If the women I interviewed hated the idea of heterosexual men sexualising their breasts, they feared being judged by women for having them visible even more. According to a study on Twitter, women used the words 'slut', 'rape', and 'whore' almost as frequently as men to slut-shame online (94,546 times for women, against 116,530 times for men).[13] Researchers Sue Jackson and Tina Vares explain that the term 'slut' has historically been used by women to talk about other women they wanted to dissociate from:

> It commonly was a way of maintaining or enforcing sexual norms. (…) For teenage girls, in particular, the term is used to brand and exclude other girls. In this instance, the 'slut' provides a strategy for the girls to carefully separate their subjectivity from the 'sluts' they watch.[14]

This description seems to be a reality for the women I interviewed, as almost all said women's judgement could be harsher. For example, when I asked Lucie how she felt about people noticing her breasts, she said that she would dread people's gaze on her body. 'I don't like them being visible, and people thinking, "Oh, look, her breasts are showing", or even getting some staring looks from men enjoying themselves and women judging and thinking, "What the fuck is this one doing?"'[15] This perception has been confirmed. Among all the age groups I interviewed, only the ones aged between 18 and 20 and between 46 and 60 did not blame women for wearing something they would consider indecent – if they did. Instead, they blamed the culture these women grew up in and the unconscious norms they had internalised. On the opposite, the other age

groups tended to assume that women wore revealing clothing to con-
sciously attract male attention.

Some participants used the word 'competition' when discussing the
'decency war' between women. For example, Tara explained how jealousy
and rivalry are an essential part of women's interactions:

> Women are so mean sometimes. So, I often prefer hearing guys talking about me
> because, at least, it would be positive most of the time, but women are just trying to
> bring each other down. It is even worse when they are jealous of a prettier girl; they
> will bring her down at all costs. It is almost a competition for men's attention: who
> is the prettiest, the sexiest?[16]

Social media users, especially Tiktok, have made fun of this competition
between women and have named that concept: a 'pick me' girl.[17] 'Pick
me' girls are described as women who try to separate themselves from
'other women' while trying to fit the definition of a 'respectable' woman
according to the male gaze. Based on examples given in an article about
these girls, when it comes to breasts, a 'pick me' could bring another
woman down for not wearing a bra and comment: 'Oh, you don't wear a
bra? I could not expose my nipples to all the men like this.'[18] Through this
behaviour, the person making the statement first shames another woman
for how she dresses while implying that she is indecent because her breasts
are heterosexual men's property. Second, this creates a sense of rivalry between the two women, as one is being openly criticised for not fitting
the norm so the other appears more 'respectable'. One of the participants,
Noa, explained how women tend to bring each other down this way:

> There are always some comments like 'Look at this one', as if there was a competition
> for the male gaze if they want to attract someone, for example. A girl could tell you
> to 'be careful with your cleavage' because they know they don't have one like yours.[19]

Lucie shares the same opinion, adding that every time she has been criticised for her clothes or body, it has been by other women. Finally, Andréa,
who is from the 50 to 60 age group, also says she experienced the same
thing. 'Women will make you understand that you are almost "dirty" or
"impure" for having your nipples visible,' she says.[20]

However, women are not shaming other women because they want to be mean to each other, but because of internalised misogyny. Internalised misogyny 'occurs when women apply sexist messages heard throughout their lives to themselves and other women'.[21] According to Alison Winch's study 'The girlfriend gaze', she describes internalised misogyny as 'women's complicity in their own disempowerment'.[22] So, even if women who slut-shame others think that they are punishing women who do not fit the norm, they are actually reinforcing gender stereotypes and limiting all women's freedom to dress and behave as they want – yes, they are actually playing against their own team.[23] Nevertheless, this misogyny is primarily subconscious because women adopt 'dominant' behaviours and language terms to find their place in a patriarchal society.[24] As Sophie Mol describes, 'Women are pushed to judge each other by rejecting the ones considered indecent.'[25] This is where the phenomenon I call 'internalised decency' happens, for example. Some women objectify themselves and learn early on that they are 'tempting sexual objects', so they internalise the idea that they must do something about it. Western societies – among others – serve them the answer on a golden plate: they need to hide their bodies. The more their brain associate 'trying to not be seen as an object' with 'covering their bodies', the more they internalise decency norms. Throughout this research, some of my participants demonstrated that they have internalised these rules. Therefore, the only way for them to not be seen as sexual objects was to be 'respectable enough' to exist as something else.

Overall, some women may feel the need to distance themselves from the stereotype of the 'slut' by putting down other women. By doing so, they signal that they are 'not like the other girls' and belong to the 're-spectable' category. Not wearing a bra is often considered a violation of decency norms. However, women may engage in slut-shaming because they have internalised the misogynistic messages they have been exposed to throughout their lives, including the objectification of women in media. This internalised misogyny can lead to the development of internalised decency as a coping mechanism to exist as something other than a sexual object. Although this behaviour limits the freedom of all women to dress as they please, it is an attitude that some women have adopted to fit into a patriarchal society that objectifies them.

2/ Good girls don't tease

Sixty per cent of women agree that they would consider it inappropriate to see another woman come into work without a bra.[26] This standard is not limited to workplaces as French schools are even stricter and do not allow bras even to be visible at all. Yes, you read it correctly. Women are held to unrealistic standards on how to cover their bodies and even how they hide their bras.

Make it look natural

Women's reputation is not solely based on whether they wear a bra; they also need to ensure that their bra is not visible. Several social rules dictate how bras are worn.[27] For example, its colour must be invisible under the woman's clothes, and the straps should not be visible. The shape must also be as smooth as possible to prevent others from guessing that the woman is wearing it to 'correct' her nipple shape.[28] While these may seem like minor details, violating these rules is seen as going against the concept of modesty, intrinsically linked with decency.[29] In his research on women's experiences of getting their first bra, Ian Brodie found that regardless of how women wear their bras, it will always communicate something to their peers and the general public: 'Bras worn when breast size does not require one communicates "something," just as not wearing a bra when one would be justified in wearing it communicates "something else".'[30] Brodie notes that even decisions of style and colour made by a woman regarding her underwear will be judged and used to categorise her.

Before the 1960s, bra straps had to remain entirely hidden, using a button sewn inside the cloth.[31] But, thanks to designers like Vivienne Westwood and Jean-Paul Gautier, bras have become less sexual and more visible, while straps slowly appear in the public sphere.[32] However, French women still consider choosing the right colour for their underwear important and often linked to their sexual reputation. Nude, pastel, light, and whitish colours are preferred because they are discreet and do not draw attention. On the other hand, colours like red or pink are considered 'too bold' and go against decency norms.[33] As Aurélia Mardon explains:

> Colour is a symbol of sexual maturity. Therefore, the woman is expected to use these objects to maintain a sexual life as a strategy of seduction within the relationship, opposite to the light colours associated with young girls, purity and virginity.[34]

Moreover, bright colours are often associated with excessive seduction and attributed to prostitutes who are 'dressed to be noticed'.[35] However, some colours are highly nuanced socially. For example, the colour Bordeaux is associated with seduction only when red is perceived as a 'dirty red'. When researchers ask young girls why they don't wear red, they explain that it is associated with being 'an easy girl'. It appears vulgar to them because it feels like 'wanting to be noticed'.[36] However, young girls must follow stricter rules than adult women, as theirs are officially written down. In French middle and high schools, a dress code is distributed at the beginning of each year. It contains many more forbidden clothing items for girls than boys.[37] For example, in some schools, girls cannot come with their legs showing or in a crop top. In almost every school, it is forbidden for girls to have their bra straps or nipples visible. In fact, even if only the straps are showing, girls could be punished for displaying 'their bra'.[38] To justify these sexist dress codes to parents complaining, some schools explain that it is 'disturbing for the boys of the school'.[39] When I asked Clara, one of my participants, her opinion on these rules, she answered: 'I think that the people who created these rules are obviously male because if you're asking for bra straps to be invisible, you must have clearly never worn one in your entire life.'[40] Noa talked about the need for French society to regulate only women's bodies:

> It makes women feel guilty. Again, it makes us return to this problem with women's rights because women's bodies are constantly debated, but men's one never. You'll never say to a man, 'Oh, your t-shirt is too transparent', or 'Why are you wearing a tank top? Your straps are showing.'[41]

The polling institute IFOP researched what items of clothing usually worn by girls French people would allow in schools.[42] The 'no bra' was forbidden by 66% of French people, and cleavage was forbidden by 62%. However, 78% said they would favour letting girls show their bra straps.[43] The mother of a French girl who was sanctioned for wearing a tank top where her bra straps were visible wrote about the objectification going into these rules:

> So far, I have not thought it necessary to question these rules aimed more at stigmatizing young women than protecting them. Protect them from who? Boys their age with whom they go to the beach, to the swimming pool (even in middle school, in mixed classes), to the gyms, on vacation, on weekends, by bus, surfing, hiking, to the cinema, to ride a bike? I imagine not. Men working in schools, then? I dare to hope not. From whom, then? We agree. It's not about protecting our young teenage girls.[44]

More than sexualising their bodies from a young age, these rules also make girls internalise decency norms. They understand that some of their body parts are so indecent that they will be punished if they display them. Later, they may carry these restrictions into adulthood and impose them on other women. As one of my participants, aged 50, Sarah, observes, 'The problem is that we expect girls to hide their breasts instead of educating men.'[45]

'A little modesty!'

In 2000, several French teen magazines were released, influencing young girls' lives. For example, *Miss, Julie*, or *Lolie* spoke to them with headlines like 'What cute guys want', '6 golden rules for your love story to last', or the main cover headline: 'How do you know if he is attracted to you?'[46] Imagine being a teenage girl who has been fed Disney's prince-charming love stories your entire childhood. You have been asked approximately 283 times if you have a 'lover' at school or been told by your family that 'you're so pretty that you'll have all the boys at your feet'. Now, you are lying in bed, reading the new issue of your favourite magazine, teaching you how to shave so boys can compliment your soft skin. What are you likely to internalise? Yes, you got it. That *you need to crave male validation.* Lucie, my participant, explains how all these magazines made her feel like she had something to prove:

> I had a magazine called *Lolie* for teenagers from 14 to 18, and I realised that it's because of these magazines that puberty, having a boyfriend, and fitting beauty standards are these big things. They prepare us to read *Glamour* when we grow up. Thinking about it, I didn't care about all this initially, but I found myself wanting to please men, thinking only about that. I don't think I would have thought about it myself without magazines. There is actual conditioning.[47]

Magazines for teenage girls started transforming the image of young girls in the 2000s until they eventually created the 'Lolita' character. This hypersexualised version of girls was mainly boosted by the rise of the beauty industry and the increasing over-sexualisation in the media.[48]

However, while magazines can condition girls to crave male approval, they also pressure them to do so correctly. A French researcher surveyed teenage magazines for eight years and found that 'magazines organise the control of behaviours, advocating for audacity, but especially etiquette, decency, and modesty'.[49] The researcher explains that women are expected to find the right balance between the erotic dimension of their appearance and being 'classy enough'. According to magazines, especially, they must master how to appear sexy without being vulgar. Otherwise, they are told that they will be despised. Girls who fail to find the right balance are usually called ' "whores" and other "sluts" or "bitches", according to the vocabulary used in magazines and among young people'.[50] While reading these magazines, young girls quickly internalise the rules and learn how to avoid being stigmatised.

Magazines were not the only ones promoting internalised decency for young girls. A famous book called *Le Dico des filles* (the girls' dictionary) was first released in 2002 and re-edited every year after that point. Inside, each page taught girls aged 12 to 16 how to behave and dress.[51] This book collection was one of the most famous in France, with more than one million books sold in 2014, and it is still being published yearly.[52] These books have been written by Dominique-Alice Rouyer, who has been clear about her faith in Christianity.[53] She clarified the values and principles she wanted to share when her books became controversial in 2014. For example, in the 'breasts' category, the author writes: 'You cannot behave like a little girl anymore. Displaying a provocative cleavage will likely attract a lot of boys around you but also some behaviours and gestures that will make you feel ashamed.'[54] This extract normalises women being harassed and slut-shamed because they 'chose' to display their breasts. The author also advises girls to 'keep being girls' when around boys, adding that 'they are not forced to act like a tomboy or a tease'.[55] This type of statement can pressure young women to internalise decency norms. It can make them feel that if they abide by those rules, they might be seen as something other than sexual objects. These books also show the link between how Christianity might influence some people's views in a way that does not benefit women's freedom. It illustrates the same kind of victim-blaming discourse some women have heard when explaining that they got sexually assaulted and blamed for it because it was believed that they had teased their rapist.[56] Therefore, girls might learn from this type of book that they should take responsibility for what happens to them if they dress in a certain way perceived as indecent.

Books, magazines, and dress codes implicitly convey to girls and women that they must not openly tease or even look like they might be doing so, even if it is just a matter of displaying their natural bodies. As a result, they internalise decency norms. Schools entirely prohibit any items of clothing where bras could be visible, which can put even more pressure on girls not to reveal their breasts or bras as it is believed to 'distract boys'. These policies reinforce decency norms from a young age. They make girls understand that they are objectified and should 'try and be something else' by hiding their bodies if they don't want to be labelled as 'sluts'.

3/ How patterns repeat themselves

But who puts pressure on young girls to dress decently first? Young girls' families, schoolmates, and social surroundings can significantly impact how they see their breasts and feel pressured by decency norms. Their close circle is usually the first socialisation experience young girls have. Therefore, these people are the ones transferring values and perceptions to them, including what they consider the norms to be. If you heard your parents tell you that you need to hide your body for years and then listened to schoolmates calling you a slut because your bra is showing, would you not internalise that your breasts are inappropriate too?

Family and sexualisation

Family members, particularly mothers, may convey internalised ideas about decency by commenting on their daughter's clothing or taking them shopping for their first bras, viewing it as a necessary step. The purchase of a first bra often begins with the realisation that 'there is a need for one', which is typically initiated by the mother or the child herself due to the comments she heard.[57] Sometimes, it is prompted by the start of breast development and the decision that they must now be covered. At other times, it is simply perceived as the girl's 'time to become a woman' due to her age, regardless of the extent of her breast development. Most of the women I interviewed reported internalising decency norms due to their mother's comments. For example, Tara admits to still feeling anxious about not wearing a bra when eating lunch with her boyfriend's parents. She adds:

> My mother always stressed me out with this when my breasts started growing. Sometimes I would display my cleavage for family meals. She would tell me that I had to hide my breasts because it was inappropriate or that it would be good not to show them so they would not be the centre of attention. So, I always had this habit of telling myself to hide them when I was with men and not to act as if I wanted to show them.[58]

Sometimes, several family members would pressure young girls not to display their breasts. Clara recounts that her parents were not the only ones checking her clothes. Her older brother also monitored her outfits before she went out. 'Once, I bought a "Friends" T-shirt when I was 17 years old, and the two cups fell precisely on my breasts. He never wanted to let me wear it.'[59]

Receiving comments like this can make young girls wonder why they were being told off for wanting to wear some clothes that were not sexualised in their eyes. For example, at 13, Tara learned that she was not allowed to be in pyjamas around men because it was too 'enticing':

> I once went to my aunt's house, where some builders worked on her terrace. I got up in the morning, wearing pyjama shorts and a loose top, and wanted breakfast on the terrace. She said to me, 'Go dress differently' I asked why, and she replied, 'Because the men are working, and you will distract them.'[60]

These comments imply that women are sexual objects and that it is better to hide them. No official teaching gives girls all the unspoken standards and rules they should follow, but the pressure is enough to teach them how to dress.[61] Lucie, one of the participants, thinks that family comments make girls understand that their bodies are becoming sexual, even though they would not see it like that initially. When asked if she sees her breasts as sexual, she answers that she does because young girls are made to understand that their breasts should be hidden. She mentions comments like 'Oh, that's it, you have to buy a bra, you have little cherries,' usually made during family gatherings. Because these comments make them uncomfortable in front of everyone, girls might feel ashamed and internalise how they need to hide. Lucie concludes that what put a lot of pressure on her was people's reactions to her breasts being visible and growing. If they did not pressure her into thinking about what 'the boys would say or think,' she would not have thought about it initially.

On the contrary, Andréa never received any comments from her family, so she never felt like she had to wear a bra to fulfil decency norms. She grew up going on holidays to the beach in Biarritz, where women used to be topless. This highlights the power that family comments can have on how young girls evolve. If women are sexualised at a young age, they might be more likely to regulate their bodies significantly and follow decency norms.

Peer pressure at school

Dress codes are not the only source of regulation for young girls at school. Their peers, who also internalised the rules, might make the same comments as their families. If children are exposed to gender stereotypes through their families, they are significantly more likely to 'punish' their schoolmates if they are not performing their gender traditionally, sometimes even excluding them based on gender.[62] Moreover, as children age and reach 9 or 10 years old, the gender stereotypes they learn slowly become morals. It is when children start to think that girls are expected to be submissive and pretty and boys to be confident and strong.[63] Finally, as they become teenagers and increasingly sexualised, children exposed to gender stereotypes are more likely to view girls as sexual objects existing to please heterosexual men and, therefore, make sexual comments about how they dress.[64] One consequence could be expecting girls to 'dress respectably' and perpetuating the social requirement for a bra.[65] Therefore, young girls' stress about hiding their breasts might increase because their surroundings – family and classmates – tell them to do so. However, sometimes it goes further than simple comments and becomes bullying. For example, Lucie argues that middle school was the worst period for her because she did not fit the norms:

> Breasts develop in middle school, where everyone scrutinises what everyone else is doing. I remember hearing things like, 'Oh hey, did you see that one? Her nipples point', and that's when you think, 'shit, what's going on?' I understood that others perceived it as an erection when it was due to many other reasons. So, I think we eventually ended up thinking it was sexual.[66]

Lucie also remembers being pressured to sexualise herself by other girls at her school. One day when she arrived, two girls from her class had made her a to-do list to follow to be more 'feminine' and attract boys. Lucie recounts that on the list were things like 'wear thongs' or 'wear a push-up bra' despite her being 11 years old. 'I was not at all into seducing boys and did not ask for any of this, but these girls planned to dress and do their hair in a way that guys might like,' she explains.[67] Éléana also remembers her schoolmates being mean to her; 'I was at school, and a girl came up to me saying, "You're not wearing a bra." I nodded, and she walked away, commenting, "It shows." '[68] She was told that people were gossiping about her because they could see her breasts moving, but Éléana never understood why they had to be still. 'When someone comments on us, we feel really embarrassed, like we've done something wrong,' she finishes.[69]

Because of these types of comments from their schoolmates, parents, and other factors developed previously, such as economic interest or purity culture, girls can internalise decency norms from a young age. These patterns are repeated, while young girls feel pressured to be decent without, most of the time, understanding why they must.

Large-breasted and inspected

Large breasts are 'rarely seen as belonging to women themselves'.[70] In Western cultures, they are linked with sexual availability and loose sexual morals. People with large breasts are considered 'incompetent, unintelligent and immodest'.[71] Regarding decency, large-breasted women are almost automatically in the wrong: their breasts are visible and cannot be hidden. These women do not have a choice. They cannot simply choose to keep their breasts 'private' while making them invisible publicly. Therefore, society makes them pay the price of something they did not even desire. Researcher Susan Brownmiller explains: 'Although they are housed on her person, from the moment they begin to show, a female discovers that her breasts are claimed by others.'[72] Parents and other family members comment on them, girlfriends compare theirs, classmates mock or take notice, and later in their lives, a partner or a baby share the 'property'. According to Brownmiller, 'no other part of the human anatomy has such semi-public, intensely private status, and no other part of the body has such vaguely defined custodial rights'.

Women can sometimes even be defined by their large breasts.[73] Tara was one of the firsts at her school to develop breasts; at 13, she was already large-breasted. She explains how hard it was for her to navigate school because of it:

During breaks, boys would pull my top to look at my breasts or touch them without my consent while I was fixing my hair bun. I read my diary from when I was 12 and found this sentence: 'Wadi asked me if he could touch my breasts today because they are big.'[74]

At the age of 14, Tara's large breasts became the defining feature people used to refer to her. They would usually say, 'It's Tara, the one with the big boobs.' Being over-sexualised at such a young age without her consent has led her to develop a negative relationship with her breasts. Clara also experienced a similar situation in school when her breasts began developing earlier than her friends. She started feeling uncomfortable with the attention boys were giving her and asked to buy her first bra. Later, when she turned 12, boys weren't talking to her anymore; they were talking to her breasts. I found that the women who had been sexualised at a young age and set the strictest clothing rules for themselves were typically those with large breasts.

Breast size is often socially linked to sexuality. Studies have shown that larger breasts are associated with a superior sexual appetite.[75] Additionally, if large-breasted women do not 'at least' attempt to conceal their breasts, they are often categorised as sexual objects.[76] One of my participants, Emma, explained that she avoids wearing colourful clothing when going out because it would draw attention to her body:

R   What clothes do you not allow yourself to wear because you feel like it would be indecent?
E   Anything that is too close to the body, anything transparent, and I am usually dressed in black every single day.
R   Why?
E   Because it is unnoticeable. If you are dressed in all black, you can't be seen. It is a way to hide. I don't want anyone commenting on my body or my breasts in the street. I just don't want to be seen.[77]

Large-breasted women are often scrutinised by the male gaze with degrading comments and intrusive stares. As a result, women often try to make their bodies unobtrusive.[78] Tara feels this urge to hide her body as well. She avoids showing her cleavage or sometimes wears loose clothing even if it is warm outside because she does not want people to see her wearing a tight or low-cut top. After hearing so many comments about her breasts and being told to hide them, she cannot imagine people in public not judging her.

Conclusion

French women seem to compete against each other for the male gaze, with some women bringing down others by pointing out what could make them 'less respectable' and 'sluttier' based on decency norms. For example, not wearing a bra or wearing flashy and 'bold' colours may be considered indecent and criticised by other women. However, women are not only scrutinised by strangers but also by their own families. Their mothers may sexualise their breasts and make them feel inappropriate if uncovered. Their schoolmates may perpetuate misogynistic patterns and decency norms learned from their parents and the world around them. Because of all this pressure and stereotypes surrounding women, young girls feel compelled to hide their breasts from a young age and internalise what they should or should not wear. Finally, large-breasted women may experience a high level of self-consciousness as this 'indecent' body part is impossible for them to conceal. As a result, these girls might grow up fearing the judgement of others, realising they cannot fit decency norms and have been treated as 'inappropriate sexual objects' since childhood.

Conclusion

While comparing women's perceptions of decency across different generations in Paris, I found that bras are mainly associated with hiding breasts and being decent by being unnoticeable. Academic research has shown that decency is linked to various factors such as religion, economy, politics, or social phenomena like internalised misogyny and patriarchy. Throughout this book, I developed the concept of 'internalised decency' – women's internalised decency norms – to show how intertwined it is with many topics. Internalised decency answers the core question of this research: *how do bras participate in making breasts indecent*? – The answer is that bras are the primary tool of internalised decency.

Bras have been around for centuries and slowly became fetishised and erotic. Capitalism and Christianity have had the most significant impact on women's breasts. Capitalism created a need for women to keep wearing bras because manufacturers could profit from them. At the same time, Christianity used bras to hide women's bodies since they urged them to dress modestly. In both cases, women were perceived as sexual objects and told to wear a bra not to tempt men, or to only wear sexy lingerie to satisfy their male partners. Bras are seen as a cover and as a sexual item simultaneously. This private versus public use of bras makes women understand that they must only display their breasts to their partner but still look enticing at home. For a few decades, in Western countries such as France, women have faced the challenge of also striking a delicate balance in public spaces. They must strive to appear 'attractive enough' while simultaneously concealing their bodies and breasts so that only their partner can appreciate what others cannot see. Women who are deemed 'sexy' are shamed and judged as much as those who are labelled 'prudish'. This oppressive societal pressure leaves no room for women to make a choice without facing criticism. To be deemed 'respectable', they must find the elusive perfect balance on the spectrum.

Women internalise misogyny and decency norms and perceive themselves as sexual objects that they need to restrict if they want to exist as anything else. Because of internalised decency, women regulate how they display their breasts and how other women display theirs. They might start judging each other's bodies, expecting breasts to be hidden to be 'respectable' and rejecting any clothing that could symbolise sexual availability. Women might internalise the difference between 'the mother and the slut' and learn to belong to the 'right' category throughout their lives.

Internalised decency also impacts women's perceptions of their bodies because they have been told that what is decent also fits beauty standards: having round, high, large but not too large breasts, and most importantly, a smooth shape. Beauty standards are responsible for women like Tara feeling like she cannot eat without a bra with her boyfriend's parents because otherwise, she would feel like her large breasts would be 'too much' and inappropriate at the table. They are also responsible for women who mention that they cannot go out with their nipples visible because other women would think that it looks 'dirty'. Nipples have a specific place in decency norms. They must be invisible to fit standards created by brands like *Dim,* who even started offering 'imperfection-correcting' bras for teenagers. Nipples are the one feature that particularly needs to be hidden because they are the main sign that a woman is not wearing a bra, and doing so might be perceived as trying to entice men. Otherwise, as Éléana explained, people would say the woman's *whole breast* is visible.

To help you understand clearly how internalised decency might be impacting your life or the lives of the women around you, I have used many scenarios described by the women in this project:

> Internalised decency happens when women think they must show their bodies to only one man because Western societies condition them to be defined and owned by the male gaze.

> Internalised decency happens when women compete with each other to be 'the right type of woman' in the eyes of men.

Internalised decency happens when people use the norms to justify behaviours like slut-shaming or harassment.

Internalised decency happens when women think they should not display their breasts if they do not naturally conform to the ideal of being round, high, perfect size, and with a smooth shape.

Internalised decency happens when young girls hear comments from their families or peers and read books and magazines mentioning their breasts, objectifying and shaming them for showing too much skin or going out without a bra.

Internalised decency happens when someone suggests that a specific type of clothes can only be worn with and for your partner if you are in a relationship.

Internalised decency happens when wearing typically deemed 'sexy' underwear and them being visible automatically puts you in the 'slut' category.

Finally, internalised decency happens when women feel more protected wearing a bra in the street because they would be less noticeable.

This list is not exhaustive, but it summarises some of the topics covered in this book. Decency rules vary from country to country and do not affect all women in the same way. However, no matter the norms they must follow, all women experiencing internalised decency are undoubtedly oppressed and monitored.

I am aware that many women around the world love wearing a bra because it provides them the support they need to get through their day. Some absolutely adore lingerie and find it beautiful, while others might appreciate the sense of 'femininity' it can make them feel. Some women may feel the pressure to wear a bra but not want to fight it. That's perfectly okay. The goal of this book is not to make you think, 'I don't want to/can't stop wearing a bra, so I'm not a feminist,' but rather to provide you with insights and awareness about how women have been conditioned to wear bras to be decent. My aim is to help you understand this piece of clothing you might wear every day and to empower you in your choice to wear it or not, especially if you feel pressured to do so.

Another important aspect I address in this book is the societal pressure that leaves women feeling hopeless and afraid of being labelled 'too sexual' or 'too prudish'. The only solution to fight this pressure is by unlearning decency norms, regardless of how you decide to do so. Women should not be pressured to dress in any way. They do not need to be 'sexy enough' or 'respectable enough'; they simply need to be allowed to make their own choices. Decency norms have been created to restrict you, but they cannot do so if you understand the origins of this oppression. Being aware of the reasons behind certain judgements and their harmful effects on women can help break patterns passed down from generation to generation. Therefore, I would like to conclude this book by thanking you, because by reading it, you are already breaking the cycle.

Notes

Introduction

1   *Le boom du 'No Bra', tendance de fond ou effet de mode ?* (2020), *IFOP*, <https://www.ifop.com/publication/le-boom-du-no-bra-tendance-de-fond-ou-effet-de-mode/> [accessed 12 July 2022].

2   Victoria Pitts-Taylor, ed., 'Cultural History of the Breast', in *Cultural Encyclopaedia of the Body [2 Volumes]* (Westport, CT: Greenwood Press, 2008), 42.

3   Claire-Lise Gaillard, *Jean-Claude Bologne Histoire de la pudeur* (n.d.), *Sentiment et modernité* <https://sentiment.hypotheses.org/84> [accessed 18 September 2022].

4   Fields, p. 2.

5   Lola Gonzalez-Quijano, 'Bologne Jean-Claude, Pudeurs féminines. Voilées, dévoilées, révélées', *Genre sexualité & société* (2011) <https://journals.openedition.org/gss/1918> [accessed 18 September 2022].

6   Matthieu Foucher, *Où en sont les études de genre en France ?* (2019), *Les Inrocks* <https://www.lesinrocks.com/actu/ou-en-sont-les-etudes-de-genre-en-france-180570-12-09-2019/> [accessed 26 September 2022].

7   Nick Inman, *The Complex History of Love, Sex and the French* (2021) <https://www.connexionfrance.com> <https://www.connexionfrance.com/article/Mag/Culture/The-complex-history-of-love-sex-and-the-French> [accessed 15 September 2022].

8   Not their real names. Views shared anonymously with their consent.

9   Maxine Craig, *Ain't I a Beauty Queen?: Culture, Social Movements, and the Politics of Race* (New York: Oxford University Press, 2002).

10 Shayne Lee, *Erotic Revolutionaries: Black Women, Sexuality, and Popular Culture* (Lanham, MD: Hamilton Books, 2010).

The making of the indecent breast

1   Victoria Bateman, *Naked Feminism: Breaking the Cult of Female Modesty* (Oxford: Polity Press, 2023), 130.
2   Ibid.
3   Ibid.
4   Pitts-Taylor, p. 37.
5   Kevin Mummey and Kathryn Reyerson, 'Whose City Is This? Hucksters, Domestic Servants, Wet-Nurses, Prostitutes, and Slaves in Late Medieval Western Mediterranean Urban Society: Whose City Is This?', *History Compass* 9, no. 12 (2011): 910–22.
6   Andrea O'Reilly, 'Wet Nursing', in *Encyclopaedia of Motherhood*, ed. Andrea O'Reilly (Thousand Oaks, CA: SAGE Publications, 2010), 1272–3.
7   Emily E. Stevens, Thelma E. Patrick, and Rita Pickler, 'A History of Infant Feeding', *The Journal of Perinatal Education* 18, no. 2 (2009): 32–9.
8   Pitts-Taylor, p. 35.
9   *Le boom du « No Bra », tendance de fond ou effet de mode ?* (2020), *IFOP*, <https://www.ifop.com/publication/le-boom-du-no-bra-tendance-de-fond-ou-effet-de-mode/> [accessed 12 July 2022].
10 Angelique Chrisafis, *French PM Suggests Naked Breasts Represent France Better than a Headscarf* (2016), *The Guardian* <https://amp.theguardian.com/world/2016/aug/30/france-manuel-valls-breasts-headscarf-burkini-ban-row> [accessed 10 July 2022].
11 Catriona Fisk, *A Decent Woman? The Breastfeeding and Visibility Debate Is Nothing New* (2016), *The Conversation* <http://theconversation.com/a-decent-woman-the-breastfeeding-and-visibility-debate-is-nothing-new-57728> [accessed 30 June 2022].
12 Ibid.
13 Pitts-Taylor, p. 36.
14 Yuliana Zaikman and Amy E. Houlihan, 'It's Just a Breast: An Examination of the Effects of Sexualization, Sexism, and Breastfeeding Familiarity on Evaluations of Public Breastfeeding', *BMC Pregnancy and Childbirth* 22, no. 1 (2022): 122.
15 Sigmund Freud, 'Female Sexuality', in *The Future of an Illusion, Civilization and Its Discontents, and Other Works* (1931), 221–44, 236.
16 Ibid.
17 Juliet Mitchell, *Psychoanalysis and Feminism*, 2nd ed. (Harlow, England: Penguin Books, 2000).
18 Pitts-Taylor, p. 37.

19 Freud, p. 225.

20 Juliet Mitchell, *Psychoanalysis and Feminism*, 2nd ed. (Harlow, England: Penguin Books, 2000).

21 Jan Van der Putten, 'Negotiating the Great Depression: The Rise of Popular Culture and Consumerism in Early-1930s Malaya', *Journal of Southeast Asian Studies* 1 (2010): 21–45.

22 Pitts-Taylor, p. 40.

23 Ibid.

24 Ibid.

25 Pitts-Taylor, p. 41.

26 Camille Favre, 'The Pin-Up: American Eroticism and Patriotism during the Second World War', *Inflexions* 38, no. 2 (2018): 181.

27 Pitts-Taylor, p. 41.

28 Pitts-Taylor, p. 42.

29 Mary Louise Pratt, *Imperial Eyes: Travel Writing and Transculturation* (Routledge, 1992), 219.

30 Ibid., p. 7.

31 Jan Riordan and Betty Ann Countryman, 'Part I: Infant Feeding Patterns Past and Present', *JOGN Nursing; Journal of Obstetric, Gynecologic, and Neonatal Nursing* 9, no. 4 (1980): 207.

32 Viv Groskop, *Not Your Mother's Milk* (2007), *The Guardian* <https://amp.theguardian.com/society/2007/jan/05/health.medicineandhealth> [accessed 29 June 2022].

33 Nicoletta Iacovidou, 'Breastfeeding in Public: A Global Review of Different Attitudes towards It', *Journal of Paediatrics & Neonatal Care* 1, no. 6 (2014).

34 Céline Hussonnois-Alaya, 'On doit se cacher': *l'allaitement en public est-il encore tabou?* (2021), *BFMTV* <https://www.bfmtv.com/societe/on-doit-se-cacher-l-allaitement-en-public-est-il-encore-tabou_AN-202110030005.html> [accessed 30 June 2022].

35 Fisk, *A Decent Woman? The Breastfeeding and Visibility Debate Is Nothing New*.

36 *Population française selon la religion France*, (2020), *Statista* <https://fr.statista.com/statistiques/472017/population-religion-france/> [accessed 12 July 2022].

37 Bateman, p. 36.

38 Bateman, p. 94.

39 Mati Meyer, *Art: Representation of Biblical Women* (n.d.), *Jewish Women's Archive*. <https://jwa.org/encyclopedia/article/art-representation-of-biblical-women> [accessed 12 July 2022].

40 Joshua J. Mark, *Women in the Middle Ages* (2019), *World History Encyclopedia*. <https://www.worldhistory.org/article/1345/women-in-the-middle-ages/> [accessed 12 July 2022].

41 Mark, *Women in the Middle Ages*.

42   The Bible. *New International Version* (1 Timothy 2:9–15).
43   Christopher P. Jones, *Why the Virgin Mary's Bare Breast Caused a Problem for Artists* (2022), *Thinksheet* <https://medium.com/thinksheet/the-artistic-problem-with-the-virgin-marys-bare-breast-19e3d4339008> [accessed 9 July 2022].
44   Pitts-Taylor, p. 36.
45   Jones, *Why the Virgin Mary's Bare Breast Caused a Problem for Artists*.
46   *What Is Purity Culture?* (2019), *Linda Kay Klein* <https://lindakayklein.com/what-is-purity-culture/> [accessed 12 July 2022].
47   Marie De Rasse, 'Vêtement féminin et pudeur. L'exemple parisien, XIVe-XVe siècles', *Hypothèses* 13, no. 1 (2010): 119–28, 122.
48   Ibid, p. 122.
49   Ibid, p. 124.
50   Jill Fields, *An Intimate Affair: Women, Lingerie, and Sexuality* (Berkeley: University of California Press, 2007), 30.
51   *Global Trends in Religiosity and Atheism 1980 to 2020* (2020), *Colin Mathers* <https://colinmathers.com/2020/09/30/global-trends-in-religiosity-and-atheism-1980-to-2020/> [accessed 12 July 2022].
52   Cavan Sieczkowski, *Pat Robertson Blames 'Awful Looking' Women for Marital Problems* (2013), *HuffPost UK* <https://www.huffpost.com/entry/pat-robertson-blames-awful-looking-women-marriage-problems_n_2479459> [accessed 11 July 2022].
53   Kristen Rosser, *Christianity and the 'Male Gaze'* (2013), *Wordgazer's Words* <http://krwordgazer.blogspot.com/2013/07/christianity-and-male-gaze.html> [accessed 11 July 2022].
54   Michelle Zancarini-Fournel, 'Genre et politique : les années 1968', *Vingtieme siecle* 75, no. 3 (2002): 133.
55   Hannah Sparks, *Pastor Slammed for Telling Wives to 'Lose Weight,' Look Less 'Butch'* (2021), *New York Post* <https://nypost.com/2021/03/03/pastor-slammed-for-telling-wives-to-lose-weight-look-less-butch/> [accessed 11 July 2022].
56   Ruth Everhart, *Who's Responsible for the Male Gaze?* (2021), *Ruth Everhart* <https://rutheverhart.com/stewart-allen-clark-preacher-whos-responsible-for-the-male-gaze/> [accessed 11 July 2022].
57   Marie De Rasse, p. 127.
58   Emma Tarlo, *Visibly Muslim: Fashion, Politics, Faith* (London, England: Bloomsbury Academic, 2010).
59   Ibid.
60   CNEWS, 'Hijab, voile, Burqa : de quoi parle-t-on et que dit la loi ?' (2021), *CNews*, <https://www.cnews.fr/france/2021-11-03/hijab-voile-burqa-de-quoi-parle-t-et-que-dit-la-loi-737077> [accessed 8 August 2023].
61   Fields, p. 3.
62   Ibid.

63 Barbara Marty, *À l'origine du soutien-gorge : une féministe révolutionnaire* (2020), *France Culture* <https://www.radiofrance.fr/franceculture/a-l-origine-du-soutien-gorge-une-feministe-revolutionnaire-1187756> [accessed 15 July 2022].

64 Simone de Beauvoir, *The Second Sex* (New York: Knopf, 1953), 189–90.

65 Fields, p. 76.

66 Angela King, 'The Prisoner of Gender: Foucault and the Disciplining of the Female Body', *Journal of International Women's Studies* 5 (2004): 29–39.

67 Fields, p. 8.

68 Marty, *À l'origine du soutien-gorge : une féministe révolutionnaire.*

69 Fields, p. 89.

70 Ibid., p. 92.

71 Ibid., p. 93.

72 Ibid., p. 96.

73 Ibid.

74 Ibid., p. 97.

75 Ibid., p. 105.

76 Ibid., p. 112.

77 Marie-Noël Boutin-Arnaud and Sandrine Tasmadjian, *Le vêtement* (Paris : Éditions Nathan, 1997), 159.

78 Delphine Martin, *Le soutien-gorge : une invention bourguignonne* (2018), *France Bleu* <https://www.francebleu.fr/infos/societe/le-soutien-gorge-une-invention-bourguignonne-1520016016> [accessed 8 August 2022].

79 Angelique Chrisafis, *France Falls Out of Love with Topless Sunbathing* (2009), *The Guardian* <https://amp.theguardian.com/lifeandstyle/2009/jul/22/topless-bathing-france> [accessed 16 July 2022].

80 Émilie Torgemen, *Pourquoi les Françaises sont de moins en moins adeptes du topless* (2019), *Le Parisien* <https://www.leparisien.fr/societe/pourquoi-les-francaises-sont-de-moins-en-moins-adeptes-du-topless-24-07-2019-8122524.php> [accessed 11 August 2022].

81 Geoff Ho, *Wonderbra: Hello Sexism, Cry Feminists* (2018), *Daily Express* <https://www.express.co.uk/life-style/life/1053249/wonderbra-adverts-hello-boys-sexism-feminism> [accessed 16 July 2022].

82 Maude Bass-Krueger, *L'histoire du soutien-gorge : tout ce que vous devez savoir sur le sous-vêtement féminin* (2019), *Vogue France* <https://www.vogue.fr/mode/article/histoire-du-soutien-gorge> [accessed 16 July 2022].

83 Bass-Krueger, *L'histoire du soutien-gorge : tout ce que vous devez savoir sur le sous-vêtement féminin.*

84 Judith Lussier, *Un symbole d'oppression* (2019), *Journal Métro* <https://journalmetro.com/actualites/national/2302827/un-symbole-doppression/> [accessed 16 July 2022].

Why are you so provocative?

1   Angela King, 'The Prisoner of Gender: Foucault and the Disciplining of the Female Body', *Journal of International Women's Studies* 5 (2004): 29–39, 34.

2   Laura Mulvey, ed., 'Visual Pleasure and Narrative Cinema', in *Visual and Other Pleasures*, 2nd ed. (Houndmills, Basingstoke, Hampshire, England/ New York: Palgrave Macmillan, 2009), 14–30.

3   Slate, *The Tragic Story behind Victoria's Secret* (2013), *HuffPost* <https://www. huffpost.com/entry/victorias-secret_n_4181683> [accessed 30 July 2022].

4   Poppy Chantler, *An Investigation Into Women's Changing Attitudes Towards Lingerie* (2019) <https://books.google.co.uk/books/about/An_Investigation_ Into_Women_s_Changing_A.html?id=LlvczQEACAAJ&redir_esc=y> [accessed 30 July 2022].

5   Diane Ponterotto, 'Resisting the Male Gaze: Feminist Responses to the "Normatization" of the Female Body in Western Culture', *Journal of International Women's Studies* 17, no. 1 (2016): 133–51, 147.

6   Barbara L. Fredrickson and Tomi-Ann Roberts, 'Objectification Theory: Toward Understanding Women's Lived Experiences and Mental Health Risks', *Psychology of Women Quarterly* 21, no. 2 (1997): 173–206.

7   Ian Brodie,' "The Harsh Reality of Being a Woman": First Bra Experiences',*Ethnologies* 29, no. 1–2 (2008): 81–106.

8   Translated from French: 'Dans les films on en revient toujours à la femme qui enlève son soutif et ça y est. C'est l'idéal, c'est la beauté. Ça n'arrive jamais dans un film qu'une femme enlève sa culotte avant son soutien-gorge. Comme si c'était ça que tu devais montrer en premier pour prouver ta féminité.'

9   Translated from French : 'Personnellement ça me fait me sentir femme quand j'ai un beau soutif et que je me trouve sexy. Après qu'est-ce que c'est se sentir féminine à part des normes sociales?'

10 Rachel Wood, ' "You Do Act Differently When You're in It": Lingerie and Femininity',*Journal of Gender Studies* 25, no. 1 (2016): 10–23.

11 Translated from French : 'Quand on a une grosse poitrine on n'aime pas trop la montrer, mais quand on a une petite poitrine on peut le vivre très mal parce qu'on n'a pas l'impression d'être une vraie femme.'

12 Translated from French: 'Je le sentais comme une obligation, après je l'ai plus pris comme un signe de féminité. C'est la façon dont je les mets en valeur, et simplement aussi parce que je trouve que la lingerie c'est super joli. La seule chose que je ne m'impose plus ce sont les soutien-gorge rembourrés. Je mets de plus en plus de soutien-gorge sans rembourrage, je laisse juste ma poitrine telle qu'elle est, mais je ressens toujours le besoin de la couvrir.'

13   Translated from French : 'J'ai presque envie de te dire que techniquement c'est ce que ça fait quand je rentre chez moi et que je l'enlève parce que ça me fait mal. Mais c'est une manière de se cacher.'

14   Translated from French : 'Ça fait 10 ans que je suis mariée, et je me retourne toujours quand je mets mon soutien-gorge. Parfois je le mets super rapidement quand je sais qu'il va regarder.'

15   Translated from French: 'C'est le pire, c'est vraiment ça le pire. Le téton est ultra associé à la sexualisation.'

16   Pitts-Taylor, p. 42.

17   Translated from French: 'C'est plutôt une question d'où je vais'

18   Translated from French : 'Je pense que je croiserais mes bras sur ma poitrine ... Je ne serais pas très à l'aise à cause de la transparence. S'il n'y a personne dans la rue, peut être que je me dirais que ce n'est pas grave, mais s'il y a quelqu'un je ne serais pas à l'aise que cette personne les voit. Je pense que ça camoufle une poitrine. Ça gomme les tétons qui pointent, ça gomme les mouvements de balanciers.'

19   Translated from French: 'Au-delà de la grosseur du sein, à partir du moment où le téton est visible on va commencer à dire qu'on "voit ton sein" et ça va être mal vu'

20   Fields, p. 96.

21   Luna Dolezal, 'The (in)Visible Body: Feminism, Phenomenology, and the Case of Cosmetic Surgery', *Hypatia* 25, no. 2 (2010): 357–75, p. 360.

22   Michelle Zancarini-Fournel, 'Genre et politique : les années 1968', *Vingtième siècle* 75, no. 3 (2002): 133.

23   Ponterotto, p. 142.

24   Ibid.

25   Fields, p. 78.

26   Ponterotto, p. 148.

27   Ibid., p. 147.

28   Bonnie Moradi and Yu-Ping Huang, 'Objectification Theory and Psychology of Women: A Decade of Advances and Future Directions', *Psychology of Women Quarterly* 32, no. 4 (2008): 37–98, 38.

29   King, p. 36.

30   Dolezal, p. 359.

31   Sandra Lee Bartky, 'Foucault, Femininity, and the Modernization of Patriarchal Power', in *Femininity and Domination* (Routledge, 2015), 73–92.

32   Jimmie Manning, 'Paradoxes of (Im)Purity: Affirming Heteronormativity and Queering Heterosexuality in Family Discourses of Purity Pledges', *Women s Studies in Communication* 38, no. 1 (2015): 99–117.

33   Kat Rosenfield, *What's Wrong with Lingerie?* (2021), *UnHerd* <https://unherd.com/2021/06/whats-wrong-with-lingerie/> [accessed 30 July 2022].

34   Translated from French : 'Mon copain maintenant est jaloux, donc je m'habille
      différemment. Mais d'un autre côté il aime aussi que je m'habille sexy, donc je ne
      sais pas.'

35   Aurélia Mardon, 'Les femmes et la lingerie : Intimité corporelle et morale
      sexuelle', *Champ psychosomatique* 27, no. 3 (2002): 69, 76.

36   Ibid.

37   Translated from French: 'Généralement les femmes qui portent de très gros
      décolletés ou des vêtements sexy sont souvent célibataires.'

38   Ponterotto, p. 147.

39   *Ma copine se met trop en valeur sur insta* (n.d.), *Jeuxvideo.com* <https://www.jeuxvi
      deo.com/forums/42-51-59198062-2-0-1-0-ma-copine-se-met-trop-en-valeur-sur-
      insta.htm> [accessed 25 July 2022].

40   *Ma copine veut faire un insta 'fitness girl'* (n.d.), *Jeuxvideo.com* <https://www.jeuxvi
      deo.com/forums/42-78-47211584-2-0-1-0-ma-copine-veut-faire-un-insta-fitness-
      girl.htm> [accessed 25 July 2022].

41   *Planetoscope – Statistiques : Consommation de Lingerie En France* (2018), *Planetoscope.
      com*   <https://www.planetoscope.com/lamour/1762-consommation-de-lingerie-
      en-france.html> [accessed 8 August 2022].

42   *Lingerie Industry Reports: Statistics, Trend, Analysis & Market Research*
      (n.d.), *Reportlinker.com*   <https://www.reportlinker.com/ci02123/Underwear.
      html> [accessed 8 August 2022].

43   Pitts-Taylor, p. 43.

44   'Emily in Paris', Netflix, 2020, episode 3, season 1.

45   Louis Chahuneau, *Aubade, l'histoire d'une marque de lingerie … pour hommes*
      (2018), *Le Point* <https://www.lepoint.fr/societe/aubade-l-histoire-d-une-marque-
      de-lingerie-pour-hommes-27-12-2018-2282022_23.php> [accessed 4 August 2022].

46   Translated from French : 'Il y a des trucs que vous n'achetez pas pour les mettre.
      La guêpière par exemple, c'est vraiment pour plaire aux hommes, parce que ce n'est
      pas confortable du tout. Quand on regarde les pubs un peu anciennes, comme les
      leçons d'Aubade où ça parle d'attirer son regard, bah là oui franchement, on te
      faisait comprendre qu'il fallait acheter pour plaire en fait.'

47   Translated from French : 'Elle m'a toujours expliqué la sexualité d'une manière
      brutale et fausse. Quand j'étais jeune elle me disait "oh tu sais un homme, tu es juste
      là pour satisfaire ses désirs sexuels, même si tu n'as pas envie".'

48   Translated from French : 'Dans ma tête, si je voulais plaire à mon copain, j'allais
      essayer de me conformer à ce qu'il aimait mais mon corps ne m'appartenait pas,
      c'était devenu uniquement le désir de l'autre.'

49   Translated from French : 'Parfois je sais que quand je parle avec mes amies, je les
      entends dire que c'est bien quand il y a le petit côté sexy avec la lingerie. Une de mes
      amies achète de plus en plus de la lingerie parce que ça fait plaisir à son copain, et la

dernière fois on en parlait et elle me disait que ça ne lui faisait pas forcément plaisir à elle de le faire.'

50 Cynthia Hamou, *Les seins et leurs complexes : forme, taille et harmonie* (2019), *Chirurgien esthétique femme à Grenoble – Rhône Alpes* <https://doct eur-hamou.com/seins-leurs-complexes-forme-taille-harmonie> [accessed 8 August 2022].

51 Translated from French : 'Si ce n'est pas quelque chose que les hommes en envie de voir, ça ne va pas être quelque chose à montrer.'

52 Fields, p. 83.

53 *A Look at the Evolution of Lingerie Ads* (2016), Bra Doctor's Blog | Now That's Lingerie <https://blog.nowthatslingerie.com/lingerie-2/a-look-at-the-evolution-of-lingerie-ads/2016/08/08> [accessed 8 August 2022].

54 Translated from French : 'Ce sont les soutien-gorge avec lesquels je vais me sentir le mieux, même s'il faut le remettre en place toute la journée. Mais finalement c'est celui qui donne la forme ronde et qui les remonte. Quand je veux mettre un décolleté par exemple, je n'en mets vraiment pas souvent, mais si je veux en mettre un, il faut que la forme soit présentable, donc je vais mettre un push-up. J'ai fait l'effort d'en acheter des non-push up, mais je ne peux pas changer le fait que je me sentirais toujours plus sexy dans un push-ups, parce que ça ressemble à l'idéal.'

55 *Le boom du « No Bra », tendance de fond ou effet de mode ?* (2020), *IFOP* <https://www.ifop.com/publication/le-boom-du-no-bra-tendance-de-fond-ou-effet-de-mode/> [accessed 12 July 2022].

56 Amy Hunt, *Is It Bad Not to Wear a Bra? Here's the Lowdown on What Could Happen to Your Cleavage* (2020), *Woman and Home Magazine* <https://www.womandh ome.com/health-and-wellbeing/bra-health-boobs-posture-354096/> [accessed 7 August 2022].

57 Bérénice Rebufa, *Dim fait complexer les ados avec un soutien-gorge qui 'gomme les imperfections'* (2016), *Konbini* <https://www.konbini.com/archive/dim-encore-soutien-gorge/> [accessed 7 August 2022].

58 Translated from French: 'Si jamais mes seins pendent un peu trop ou si le décolleté est trop important, dans ce cas-là je vais mettre un soutien-gorge pour les faire remonter un peu plus.'

59 Translated from French: 'Les pubs c'est genre "si tu portes ce soutien-gorge, ton complexe va disparaître".'

60 Nelly Quemener, '« Ma Chérie, Il Faut Révéler Ta Féminité ! »: Rhétorique Du Choix et de l'émancipation Dans Les Émissions de Relooking En France', *Raisons Politiques* 62, no. 2 (2016): 35, 44.

61 Alyssa Baxter, 'Faux Activism in Recent Female-Empowering Advertising', *Elon Journal of Undergraduate Research in Communications* 6, no. 1 (2015). <http://www.inquiriesjournal.com/articles/1133/faux-activism-in-recent-female-empower ing-advertising> [accessed 8 August 2022].

62   Translated from French: 'Montrer qui on est'
63   Léa Drouelle, *Wonderbra tente une pub 'féministe' et se fait tacler*
     (2018), *Terrafemina* <https://www.terrafemina.com/article/sexisme-la-nouvelle-pub-wonderbra-fait-reagir_a347053/1> [accessed 7 August 2022].
64   Translated from French: 'Ça propage l'idée qu'on a besoin d'acheter quelque chose pour aimer notre corps. Ils se sont rendu compte que ça passait plus dans la société d'utiliser le sexisme donc ils ont dû trouver autre chose.'
65   Baxter, 2015.
66   Ibid.
67   Léa Drouelle, *Wonderbra tente une pub 'féministe' et se fait tacler*
     (2018), *Terrafemina* <https://www.terrafemina.com/article/sexisme-la-nouvelle-pub-wonderbra-fait-reagir_a347053/1> [accessed 7 August 2022].
68   Fields, p. 3.

Social media and objectification of women's breasts

1   Rachel Millsted and Hannah Frith, 'Being Large-Breasted: Women Negotiating Embodiment', *Women's Studies International Forum* 26, no. 5 (2003): 455–65, 456.
2   Ponterotto, p. 134.
3   Esteban Ortiz-Ospina, *The Rise of Social Media* (2019), *Our World in Data* <https://ourworldindata.org/rise-of-social-media> [accessed 7 September 2022].
4   Andrea Cardenas, *The Hypersexualization of Society* (2021), *Exploring Your Mind* <https://exploringyourmind.com/the-hypersexualization-of-society/> [accessed 18 August 2022].
5   Sonia Suarez, *Objectification and Women Empowerment: The Social Media Scene* (2021), *Engagewithscience.org* <https://engagewithscience.org/objectification-and-women-empowerment-the-social-media-scene/> [accessed 18 August 2022].
6   Annie Berry, *The Hyper-sexualization of Women in Nicki Minaj's 'Anaconda' Music Video Is Reinforcing Patriarchal Values* (2020), *Medium* <https://medium.com/@a.m.berry/the-hyper-sexualization-of-women-in-nicki-minajs-anaconda-music-video-is-reinforcing-32970f8afd7c> [accessed 18 August 2022].
7   Charles Manning, *Nicki Minaj Worries about the Impact She Has Had on Young Women* (2018), *Daily Front Row*. Available at: <https://fashionweekdaily.com/nikki-minaj-elle-cover/> [accessed 25 August 2022].
8   Berry, 2020.
9   *What Is Hypersexualization* (n.d.), *Igi-global.com* <https://www.igi-global.com/dictionary/overcoming-barriers/94467> [accessed 18 August 2022].

10   Bonnie Moradi and Yu-Ping Huang, 'Objectification Theory and Psychology of Women: A Decade of Advances and Future Directions', *Psychology of Women Quarterly* 32, no. 4 (2008): 377–98.

11   Linda Papadopoulos, *Sexualisation of Young People – Review* [eBook] (2010), Available at: <https://dera.ioe.ac.uk/10738/1/sexualisation-young-people.pdf> [accessed 26 August 2022].

12   Suarez, 2021.

13   Elizabeth A. Daniels, Eileen L. Zurbriggen, and L. Monique Ward, 'Becoming an Object: A Review of Self-Objectification in Girls', *Body Image* 33 (2020): 278–99.

14   Translated from French: 'Je suis des influenceuses et je suis horrifiée par ce que je vois. Elles hypersexualisent leurs enfants en leur mettant des hauts de maillot, des soutien-gorge alors qu'elles viennent à peine d'avoir des seins, et elles ne s'en rendent même pas compte. Le problème avec les femmes, que ce soient les soutien-gorge ou n'importe quoi d'autres, c'est que toutes les possibilités ont été créées, soit pour nous cacher, soit pour nous montrer. Et ces enfants se retrouvent hypersexualisés par leurs parents en prenant des poses telles que l'homme voudrait. Les femmes qui s'habillent d'une manière considérée "sexy", est ce que c'est une réelle liberté ou est-ce que c'est une soumission ?'

15   Translated from French : 'Quelqu'un qui porte un soutien-gorge à 8 ans, pour moi c'est de l'hypersexualisation. Mais quelqu'un de n'importe quel âge qui poste une photo sans soutien-gorge, je ne considère pas ça sexuel. L'hypersexualisation vient des adultes.'

16   Translated from French : 'Personnellement ça me dérange quand je vois que la personne essaie vraiment de les mettre en avant parce que ça donne l'impression qu'il n'y a que ça à voir chez une femme. Il y a une différence entre une personne qui va mettre quelque chose d'hyper moulant sans soutien-gorge avec un décolleté de malade et une fille qui ne met juste pas de soutien-gorge parce qu'elle s'en fout, je pense qu'on voit vraiment la différence. J'ai l'impression qu'elle se dise que pour appâter les hommes elles savent ce qu'elles doivent sortir.'

17   Translated from French : 'Ce que je vais trouver provocant c'est la volonté d'attirer. Choisir une photo où on a les tétons visibles sous un top démontre d'une envie de créer une réaction.'

18   Sarah Pruitt, *What Are the Four Waves of Feminism?* (2022), *History* <https://www.history.com/news/feminism-four-waves> [accessed 18 August 2022].

19   Olivier Peguy, *#MeToo, #Balancetonporc, trois ans après* (2020), *Euronews*. Available at: <https://fr.euronews.com/2020/10/21/metoo-balancetonporc-trois-ans-apres> [accessed 25 August 2022].

20   Ibid.

21   Pauline Chateau, *'Balance ton quoi', le nouveau clip d'Angèle (avec Pierre Niney) qui fait le procès du sexisme* (2019), *Le HuffPost*. Available at: <https://www.huffing tonpost.fr/culture/article/balance-ton-quoi-le-nouveau-clip-d-angele-avec-pierre-niney-qui-fait-le-proces-du-sexisme_143606.html> [accessed 25 August 2022].

22   Jonathan Blake, *Instagram Allows Breastfeeding and Post-Op Scars in New Guidelines* (2015), *BBC* <https://www.bbc.co.uk/news/newsbeat-32340412> [accessed 7 September 2022].

23   Gabby Bush, Mariam Nadeem, Marc Cheong, and et al., *Trump, Nipples and the Hypocrisy of the Social Media Giants* (2021), *Pursuit* (The University of Melbourne) <https://pursuit.unimelb.edu.au/articles/trump-nipples-and-the-hypocrisy-of-the-social-media-giants> [accessed 7 September 2022].

24   The New York Times, *Will Instagram ever 'free the nipple'?* (2019), *The New York Times*. Available at: <https://www.nytimes.com/2019/11/22/arts/design/instag ram-free-the-nipple.html> [accessed 19 August 2022].

25   Ibid.

26   Ibid.

27   Translated from French: 'Il y a des choses qui sont pires qui sont sur les réseaux, mais on censure les tétons. Et au final le fait qu'on censure, ça conforte la société dans le fait que ce n'est pas quelque chose de décent et que ça ne devrait pas être montré alors que les hommes ont les mêmes.'

28   Virginia Harrison, *Outrage Erupts over Facebook's Decision on Graphic Videos* (2013), *CNNMoney* <https://money.cnn.com/2013/10/22/news/companies/facebook-violent-videos/> [accessed 7 September 2022].

29   Danielle Harris, *Sexist Censorship on Social Media* (2016), *The DePaulia*. Available at: <https://depauliaonline.com/19576/opinions/censorship-free-the-nipple/> [accessed 19 August 2022].

30   Jaclyn Friedman, *What You Really Really Want: The Smart Girl's Shame-Free Guide to Sex and Safety* (Seattle, WA: Seal Press, 2011).

31   Elizabeth A. Armstrong, Laura T. Hamilton, Elizabeth M. Armstrong, and J. Lotus Seeley, ' "Good Girls": Gender, Social Class, and Slut Discourse on Campus', *Social Psychology Quarterly* 77, no. 2 (2014): 100–22.

32   Lydia Spencer-Elliott, *This Is the Story behind Janet Jackson's Super Bowl 'Wardrobe Malfunction'* (2022), *Grazia* <https://graziadaily.co.uk/life/tv-and-film/janet-jack son-documentary-timberlake-super-bowl/> [accessed 19 August 2022].

33   Ibid.

34   Pitts-Taylor, p. 41.

35   Pratt, p. 7.

36   Shayne Lee, *Erotic Revolutionaries: Black Women, Sexuality, and Popular Culture* (Lanham, MD: Hamilton Books, 2010) – See also the book *Fashion and Cultural Studies* by Susan B. Kaiser and Denise N. Green, which explores how race, ethnicity, class, and gender intersect.

37 Catherine McCormack, *Women in the Picture: Women, Art and the Power of Looking* (Basingstoke, England: Icon Books, 2021).

38 Ibid.

39 Ibid.

40 Translated from French: 'Je pense que sur les réseaux on accepte plus facilement que les filles montrent leurs corps puisque la société veut ça, mais d'un autre côté on se fait d'autant plus critiquer pour ça. Je pense que le paradoxe est beaucoup plus poussé sur les réseaux sociaux parce que dans la vie normale les gens ne vont pas trop partager leurs opinions à voix haute.'

41 Jessica Ringrose, 'Are You Sexy, Flirty, or a Slut? Exploring "Sexualization" and How Teen Girls Perform/Negotiate Digital Sexual Identity on Social Networking Sites', in *New Femininities* (London: Palgrave Macmillan UK, 2011), 99–116, 107.

42 Ibid.

43 Translated from French : 'Je pense que les gens se lâchent encore plus sur les réseaux sociaux, alors que déjà dans la rue les gens sont sans filtre, mais en ligne c'est encore pire.'

44 Melissa Davey, *Online Violence against Women 'Flourishing', and Most Common on Facebook, Survey Finds* (2020), *The Guardian* <https://amp.theguardian.com/society/2020/oct/05/online-violence-against-women-flourishing-and-most-common-on-facebook-survey-finds> [accessed 19 August 2022].

45 Translated from French : 'Dans la vraie vie je sais me préparer mentalement. Je sais par où je passe, alors que sur les réseaux, n'importe qui peut prendre une capture d'écran, je ne sais pas où ça va aller. Je n'ai pas envie de me faire insulter par exemple.'

46 Manal Lyna El Euldj, and Ambre Marionneau, *'Expose-toi et tais-toi' : les femmes, premières victimes des réseaux sociaux* (2020), *Numerique-investigation.org* <https://numerique-investigation.org/la-critique-systematique-des-personnes-percues-comme-femme-sur-les-reseaux-sociaux/4847/> [accessed 22 August 2022].

47 Ibid.

48 France Info, *86% des Françaises victimes d'au moins une forme d'atteinte ou d'agression sexuelle dans la rue : un chiffre* (2018), *Franceinfo* <https://www.francetvinfo.fr/societe/harcelement-sexuel/86-des-francaises-victimes-d-au-moins-une-forme-d-atteinte-ou-dagression-sexuelle-dans-la-rue-un-chiffre-absolument-terrifiant_3042091.html> [accessed 22 August 2022].

49 Translated from French: 'Sur les réseaux tu peux le mettre en privé, alors que si je vais dans la rue tout le monde peut regarder et n'importe qui peut venir me parler.»

50 Mike Wade, *Social Media Fuels Offline Misogyny, Says Top Lawyer* (2022), *Times* <https://www.thetimes.co.uk/article/social-media-fuels-offline-misogyny-says-top-lawyer-qcpnd68sq> [accessed 22 August 2022].

51 Shanti Das, *Inside the Violent, Misogynistic World of TikTok's New Star, Andrew Tate* (2022), *The Guardian* <https://amp.theguardian.com/technology/2022/aug/06/andrew-tate-violent-misogynistic-world-of-tiktok-new-star> [accessed 22 August 2022].

52   Emma Kelly, *Andrew Tate Claims Women Should 'Bear Responsibility' for Being Raped* (2017), *Metro.co.uk* <https://metro.co.uk/2017/10/19/big-brothers-and rew-tate-says-women-should-bear-responsibility-for-being-raped-in-vile-tweets-7011756/> [accessed 22 August 2022].

53   Shanti Das, 2022.

54   Emma Kelly, *Andrew Tate: Money-Making Scheme for Fans of 'Extreme Misogynist' Closes* (2022), *The Guardian* <https://amp.theguardian.com/media/2022/aug/20/andrew-tate-money-making-scheme-for-fans-of-extreme-misogynist-closes> [accessed 22 August 2022].

55   El Euldj, Marionneau, 2020.

56   Marylène Lieber, 'Le sentiment d'insécurité des femmes dans l'espace public : une entrave à la citoyenneté ?', *Nouvelles questions féministes* 21, no. 1 (2002): 41–56.

57   Glenda Cooper, *Women Too Scared to Go Out Alone* (1997), *Independent* <https://www.independent.co.uk/news/uk/home-news/women-too-scared-to-go-out-alone-1273125.html> [accessed 7 September 2022].

58   Carol Brooks Gardner, *Passing by: Gender and Public Harassment* (Berkeley, CA: University of California Press, 1995).

59   Lieber, p. 44.

60   Ibid.

61   Translated from French : 'Si la femme n'en met pas on dira que c'était pour ça, mais si elle en met un on dira que c'était parce qu'on voyait la bretelle ou que c'était trop aguicheur. Ils trouveront toujours une excuse. On nous fait croire qu'en cachant la forme on se protège mais pas du tout.'

62   Translated from French : 'J'ai déjà eu beaucoup de situations dans le métro où la personne est juste pressée contre mes seins ou des mecs qui te disent des trucs dégueulasses dans l'oreille. Et c'est aussi pour ça que j'ai peur. Ma peur de pas mettre de soutien-gorge dans la rue elle vient de là. J'ai peur que ça se remarque plus. On est toujours plus de femmes à mettre des soutien-gorge qu'à ne pas en mettre, donc forcément ça se remarque plus, et moi je n'ai pas envie de me faire remarquer. Tout le temps regardée, jugée. On entend toujours 'ok ce n'est pas une raison pour la violer mais là quand même'. Plus il y a de couches plus je me sens protégée. Si jamais je mets une robe ou quelque chose de décolleté, je vais mettre un débardeur en dessous pour cacher le décolleté, comme ça je me sens en sécurité.'

63   Translated from French : 'Je pense que dans le harcèlement de rue, parfois on se fait moins emmerder quand on porte un soutif, mais je pense que ça ne ferait pas une grande différence, c'est plutôt psychologique je pense. Mais encore ça dépend du soutif parce que je pense que malheureusement, plus on souligne le décolleté, plus on a tendance à se sentir en danger.'

Women vs women

1   Translated from French : 'Je ne voudrais pas que des femmes pensent "mais qu'est-ce qu'elle fout celle-là"'

2   Translated from French: 'On nous dit des trucs comme "fais gaffe à ton sein qui dépasse" "on voit tes tétons" ou quoi. Au final tu dois faire attention parce que les autres pourraient te regarder.'

3   Fields, p. 138.

4   Translated from French : -Je me dis "habille toi", et que j'ai l'impression qu'on voit que ça et qu'ils pensent tous que je veux les montrer.
     -Pourquoi c'est un problème de vouloir les montrer ?
     -Ça donne une image de fille qui cherche l'attention.

5   *Le boom du « No Bra », tendance de fond ou effet de mode ?* (2020), *IFOP* <https://www.ifop.com/publication/le-boom-du-no-bra-tendance-de-fond-ou-effet-de-mode/> [accessed 12 July 2022].

6   Lady Dylan, *Je veux comprendre … le slut-shaming* (2017), *Madmoizelle* <https://www.madmoizelle.com/slut-shaming-115244> [accessed 8 September 2022].

7   Ibid.

8   Translated from French : 'Pour certains c'est toujours l'histoire de la mère et la putain, c'est toujours ce truc où on est ou l'un ou l'autre mais on ne peut pas être les deux, alors que c'est faux. On est les deux.'

9   Sophie Mol, *Le slut-shaming, cet inconnu qui vous veut du bien ?* (2017), *Uclouvain.be.* Available at: <https://dial.uclouvain.be/memoire/ucl/en/object/thesis%3A10875/datastream/PDF_01/view> [accessed 8 September 2022], p. 20.

10   Ibid.

11   Ibid.

12   Translated from French : 'Si je mets un décolleté je vais être considérée comme une pute, si je m'habille trop, je suis prude.'

13   *The Use of Misogynistic Terms on Twitter* (2016), *Demos.co.uk* <https://www.demos.co.uk/wp-content/uploads/2016/05/Misogyny-online.pdf> [accessed 9 September 2022].

14   Sue Jackson and Tina Vares, 'Media "Sluts": "Tween" Girls' Negotiations of Postfeminist Sexual Subjectivities in Popular Culture', in *New Femininities* (London: Palgrave Macmillan UK, 2011), 134–46, 139.

15   Translated from French : 'Je n'aime pas que ça soit visible et qu'on puisse se dire "ah bah tiens on voit ses seins" ou qu'il y ait des regards un peu insistants, soit des hommes qui prennent leur pied et des femmes qui jugent en se disant "mais qu'est-ce qu'elle fout celle-là".'

16   Translated from French : 'Les filles sont tellement des garces parfois. Parfois je
      me dis que je préfère entendre des mecs qui parlent de moi que des femmes parce
      qu'au moins eux c'est positif, alors qu'elles se tirent dans les pattes. C'est encore pire
      quand elles sont jalouses d'une fille qui est plus belle qu'elles, elles vont essayer de la
      descendre par tous les moyens. C'est presque comme une compétition par rapport
      aux hommes. C'est toujours celle qui est la plus belle, la plus sexy'

17   Bysoraya Johnson, *The Problem with "Pick Me" Girls* (2020), *Affinitymagazine.
      Us* <http://affinitymagazine.us/2020/06/25/the-problem-with-pick-me-girls/>
      [accessed 9 September 2022].

18   Ibid.

19   Translated from French : 'Il y a toujours des petits commentaires "regarde celle-là",
      comme s'il y avait une forme de compétition par rapport au regard de l'homme si
      on veut plaire par exemple. Une fille pourrait te dire "fais attention à ton décolleté"
      parce qu'elle sait qu'elle n'en a pas un comme ça.'

20   Translated from French : 'Les femmes vont te faire comprendre que tu es presque
      "sale" que tu es "impure" parce que tes tétons se voient'

21   Kira K. Means, ' "Not Like Other Girls": Implicit and Explicit Dimensions of
      Internalized Sexism and Behavioral Outcomes', *WWU Graduate School Collection*
      (2021).

22   Alison Winch, 'The Girlfriend Gaze', in *Girlfriends and Postfeminist
      Sisterhood* (London: Palgrave Macmillan UK, 2013), 8–32, 22.

23   Papp, Erchull, and Liss, 2017.

24   Florence Laffut and Florence Ronveaux. *Slut-shaming : un nouveau phénomène vieux
      comme le monde* (2014), *CVFE – Dire NON aux violences conjugales !* <https://
      www.cvfe.be/publications/analyses/227-slut-shaming-un-nouveau-phenomene-
      vieux-comme-le-monde> [accessed 9 September 2022].

25   Sophie Mol, *Le slut-shaming, cet inconnu qui vous veut du bien ?* (2017), *Uclouvain.
      be*. Available at: <https://dial.uclouvain.be/memoire/ucl/en/object/thesis%3A10
      875/datastream/PDF_01/view> [accessed 8 September 2022], p. 20.

26   *Le boom du « No Bra », tendance de fond ou effet de mode ?* (2020), *IFOP* <https://
      www.ifop.com/publication/le-boom-du-no-bra-tendance-de-fond-ou-effet-de-
      mode/> [accessed 12 July 2022].

27   Aurélia Mardon, 'Les femmes et la lingerie : Intimité corporelle et morale
      sexuelle', *Champ psychosomatique* 27, no. 3 (2002): 69, 70.

28   Ibid.

29   Ibid, p. 74.

30   Ian Brodie, ' "The Harsh Reality of Being a Woman": First Bra Experiences',
      Ethnologies 29, no. 1–2 (2008): 81–106, 84.

31   Mardon, p. 74.

32   Ibid.

33   Ibid.

34 Ibid., p. 74.

35 Ibid., p. 71.

36 Ibid.

37 Léa Guedj, *Dans les collèges et les lycées, tenue correcte exigée … surtout pour les filles* (2018), *France Inter* <https://www.radiofrance.fr/franceinter/dans-les-colleges-et-les-lycees-tenue-correcte-exigee-surtout-pour-les-filles-9176333> [accessed 10 September 2022].

38 Ibid.

39 Ibid.

40 Translated from French : 'Je pense que les personnes qui ont créé ces règles sont forcément des hommes déjà, parce que pour demander que des bretelles de soutien-gorge soient invisible, il faut vraiment n'avoir jamais porté de soutien-gorge de sa vie.'

41 Translated from French : 'Je trouve ça hyper culpabilisant. Et encore une fois ça ramène a cette questions des textes de loi, parce que le corps de la femme est toujours un sujet, le corps des hommes jamais. Tu ne vas jamais dire à un homme "oh ton t-shirt est trop transparent", "pourquoi tu mets un débardeur ? On voit tes bretelles.'

42 François Kraus and Louise Jussian, *POUR LES FRANCAIS, QU'EST-CE QU'UNE « TENUE CORRECTE » POUR UNE FILLE AU LYCÉE?* (2020), *Ifop.com* <https://www.ifop.com/wp-content/uploads/2020/09/Ifop_C rop_mar.top_2020.09.23.pdf> [accessed 10 September 2022].

43 Ibid., p. 3.

44 Estelle Alquier, *Couvrez cette bretelle de soutien-gorge que je ne saurais voir* (2020), *Mediapart* <https://blogs.mediapart.fr/estelle-alquier/blog/200920/couvrez-cette-bretelle-de-soutien-gorge-que-je-ne-saurais-voir> [accessed 12 September 2022].

45 Translated from French : 'En fait le problème c'est qu'on attend des filles de cacher leurs seins, plutôt que d'éduquer les hommes.'

46 Pierre Galouise, *Top 10 des magazines pour ado des années 2000 (ceux qui nous ont le plus structuré intellectuellement)* (2021), *Topito* <https://www.topito.com/top-magazine-people-2000> [accessed 10 September 2022].

47 Translated from French : ' J'avais un magazine qui s'appelait Lolie pour les ados de 14 à 18 ans, et je me suis rendu compte que c'étaient ces magazines-là qui faisait tout un truc de la puberté, d'avoir un petit copain, les standards de beauté, et qui nous préparent à lire Glamour plus tard. En y réfléchissant, je pense que je m'en foutais de tout ça, pour moi c'était juste naturel, mais j'étais très sensible à tout ça et je me suis retrouvée moi aussi à vouloir leur plaire, à penser qu'à ça, et je ne suis pas convaincue que j'y aurais pensé par moi-même. Il y a vraiment un conditionnement qui se fait.'

48   Philippe Liotard and Sandrine Jamain-Samson, 'La « Lolita » et la « sex bomb »,
     figures de socialisation des jeunes filles. L'hypersexualisation en question', *Sociologie
     et societes* 43, no. 1 (2011): 45–71, 57.
49   Ibid.
50   Ibid, p. 59.
51   *Le Dico des filles : rose toxique* (2014), *Gazette des femmes* <https://gazettedesfem
     mes.ca/9813/le-dico-des-filles-rose-toxique/> [accessed 10 September 2022].
52   Ibid.
53   Sémiramis Ide, *Le dico des filles, le top du sexisme* (2014), *Information
     TV5MONDE* <https://information.tv5monde.com/terriennes/le-dico-des-filles-
     le-top-du-sexisme-3126> [accessed 13 September 2022].
54   Lydia Menez, Margaux Ravard, and Auriane Guerithault, « *On culpabilise
     les jeunes filles dans tout l'ouvrage* » : *la rédaction a relu le « Dico des filles »*
     (2022), *ELLE* <https://www.elle.fr/Societe/News/On-culpabilise-les-jeunes-fil
     les-dans-tout-l-ouvrage-la-redaction-a-relu-le-Dico-des-filles-4021909> [accessed
     10 September 2022].
55   Ibid.
56   'Addressing Rape Culture: The Unbearable Flippancy of French Media'
     (2022), *Institut Du Genre En Géopolitique* <https://igg-geo.org/?p=8230&lang=
     en> [accessed 4 August 2023].
57   Brodie, p. 86.
58   Translated from French : 'Ma mère m'a toujours stressée avec ça quand j'ai
     commencé à avoir des seins. Parfois je mettais des décolletés pour les repas de fa-
     mille et elle me disait qu'il fallait que je les cache parce que ce n'était pas approprié
     ou que ça serait bien de pas en mettre pour que ce ne soit pas le centre de l'attention.
     J'ai toujours eu cette habitude de me dire qu'il fallait que je les cache quand j'étais
     avec des hommes pour pas agir comme si j'avais envie de les montrer.'
59   Translated from French : 'Une fois j'avais acheté un T-shirt "Friends", j'avais 17 ans,
     et les deux tasses tombaient exactement sur mes deux seins. Il n'a jamais voulu me
     laisser le porter.'
60   Translated from French : 'Une fois quand j'allais chez ma tante, j'avais 13 ans et elle
     faisait faire des travaux sur sa terrasse. Je m'étais levée le matin et j'étais en short
     de pyjama avec un haut un peu large et je voulais prendre le petit déjeuner sur la
     terrasse. Elle m'a dit "va t'habiller autrement" j'ai demandé pourquoi, et elle m'a
     répondu "parce que les hommes sont en train de travailler et tu vas les déconcentrer."'
61   Mardon, p. 70.
62   Kristen L. Granger, Laura D. Hanish, Olga Kornienko, and et al., 'Preschool
     Teachers' Facilitation of Gender-Typed and Gender-Neutral Activities during Free
     Play', *Sex Roles* 76, no. 7–8 (2017): 498–510.
63   R. W. Blum, K. Mmari, and C. Moreau, 'It Begins at 10: How Gender
     Expectations Shape Early Adolescence around the World' [online], *The Journal*

of Adolescent Health: Official Publication of the Society for Adolescent Medicine 61, 4 Suppl. (2017): S3–S4. Available at: <https://www.jahonline.org/article/S1054-139X(17)30355-5/fulltext> [accessed 20 September 2022].

64 J. Jewell, C. Spears Brown, and B. Perry, 'All My Friends Are Doing It: Potentially Offensive Sexual Behavior Perpetration within Adolescent Social Networks' [online], *Journal of Research on Adolescence: The Official Journal of the Society for Research on Adolescence* 25, no. 3 (2015): 592–604.

65 Brodie, p. 90.

66 Translated from French : 'Les seins arrive au collège là où tout le monde scrute ce que tout le monde fait. Je me souviens des réflexions comme "oh tiens tu as vu celle-là elle a les tétons qui pointent" et c'est là qu'on se dit "merde, qu'est-ce qu'il se passe?" et j'ai compris que c'était perçu par les autres un peu comme une érection, alors que c'est dû à tellement d'autres raisons. Donc je pense qu'à termes on a fini par penser que c'était quelque chose de sexuel.'

67 Translated from French: 'J'étais pas du tout dans un rapport de séduction avec les garçons et je n'avais rien demandé mais les filles qui s'organisaient entre-elles pour faire en sorte de s'habiller, se coiffer d'une manière qui pourrait leur plaire.'

68 Translated from French : 'Je me rappelle une fois être à l'école et avoir une fille qui vient me voir en me disant "tu ne portes pas de soutien-gorge," j'ai acquiescé, et elle est partie en commentant "ça se voit".'

69 Translated from French : 'Quand on nous fait une remarque on se sent vraiment gênée, comme si on avait fait quelque chose de mal.'

70 Rachel Millsted and Hannah Frith, 'Being Large-Breasted: Women Negotiating Embodiment', *Women's Studies International Forum* 26, no. 5 (2003): 455–65, 456.

71 Ibid.

72 Laurel Richardson and Susan Brownmiller, 'Femininity', *Contemporary Sociology* 14, no. 1 (1985): 80, 24.

73 Millsted and Frith, p. 458.

74 Translated from French : 'À la pause, les garçons me tiraient mon haut pour regarder mes seins ou touchaient mes seins sans mon consentement pendant que je refaisais mon chignon. J'ai relu mon journal intime de quand j'avais 12 ans récemment et j'ai trouvé une phrase 'Wadi m'a demandé s'il pouvait toucher mes seins aujourd'hui à l'école parce qu'ils sont gros.'

75 Brodie, p. 93.

76 Ibid.

77 Translated from French : 'R- Quels vêtements tu ne t'autorises pas à porter au niveau du haut de ton corps, parce que tu as l'impression que ça serait indécent ? Emma- Tout ce qui est moulant, les tops transparents et de manière générale, je m'habille tous les jours en noir. R- Pourquoi ?

E- Parce que ça passe inaperçu. Parce que si tu es habillée vraiment tout en noir, ça se voit moins. C'est une manière de se cacher. Dans la rue je n'ai pas envie qu'on me fasse de remarque sur mon corps ou ma poitrine, comme si je ne voulais pas être vue.'

78   Millsted and Frith, p. 461.

Bibliography

Websites

86% des Françaises victimes d'au moins une forme d'atteinte ou d'agression sexuelle dans rue : un chiffre (2018), *Franceinfo* <https://www.francetvinfo.fr/societe/harc element-sexuel/86-des-francaises-victimes-d-au-moins-une-forme-d-atteinte-ou-dagression-sexuelle-dans-la-rue-un-chiffre-absolument-terrifiant_3042091. html> [accessed 22 August 2022].

Alquier, Estelle. *Couvrez cette bretelle de soutien-gorge que je ne saurais voir* (2020), *Mediapart* <https://blogs.mediapart.fr/estelle-alquier/blog/200920/couv rez-cette-bretelle-de-soutien-gorge-que-je-ne-saurais-voir> [accessed 12 September 2022].

Aubade Lingerie de Femme – Le Calendrier 2000 (n.d.), *Voisin.Ch* <https://www.voi sin.ch/aubade/calendrier_2000.html> [accessed 8 August 2022].

Bass-Krueger, Maude. *L'histoire du corset : tout ce que vous devez savoir sur la pièce de lingerie culte* (2019), *Vogue France* <https://www.vogue.fr/mode/article/lhisto ire-du-corset-tout-ce-que-vous-devez-savoir-sur-la-piece-de-lingerie-culte> [accessed 15 July 2022].

——. *L'histoire du soutien-gorge : tout ce que vous devez savoir sur le sous-vêtement féminin* (2019), *Vogue France* <https://www.vogue.fr/mode/article/histoire-du-soutien-gorge> [accessed 16 July 2022].

Berry, Annie. *The Hyper-Sexualization of Women in Nicki Minaj's 'Anaconda' Music Video Is Reinforcing Patriarchal Values* (2020), *Medium* <https://medium. com/@a.m.berry/the-hyper-sexualization-of-women-in-nicki-minajs-anaco nda-music-video-is-reinforcing-32970f8afd7c> [accessed 18 August 2022].

Blake, Jonathan. *Instagram Allows Breastfeeding and Post-Op Scars in New Guidelines* (2015), *BBC* <https://www.bbc.co.uk/news/newsbeat-32340412> [accessed 7 September 2022]

Bush, Gabby, Mariam Nadeem, Marc Cheong, and et al. *Trump, Nipples and the Hypocrisy of the Social Media Giants* (2021), *Pursuit* (The University of Melbourne) <https://pursuit.unimelb.edu.au/articles/trump-nipples-and-the-hypocrisy-of-the-social-media-giants> [accessed 7 September 2022].

Cardenas, Andrea. *The Hypersexualization of Society* (2021), *Exploring Your Mind* <https://exploringyourmind.com/the-hypersexualization-of-society/> [accessed 18 August 2022].

Chahuneau, Louis. *Aubade, l'histoire d'une marque de lingerie … pour hommes* (2018), *Le Point* <https://www.lepoint.fr/societe/aubade-l-histoire-d-une-marque-de-lingerie-pour-hommes-27-12-2018-2282022_23.php> [accessed 4 August 2022].

Chantler, Poppy. *An Investigation Into Women's Changing Attitudes Towards Lingerie* (2019) <https://books.google.co.uk/books/about/An_Investigation_Into_Women_s_Changing_A.html?id=LlvczQEACAAJ&redir_esc=y> [accessed 30 July 2022].

Chateau, Pauline. *'Balance ton quoi', le nouveau clip d'Angèle (avec Pierre Niney) qui fait le procès du sexisme* (2019), *Le HuffPost*. Available at: <https://www.huffingtonpost.fr/culture/article/balance-ton-quoi-le-nouveau-clip-d-angele-avec-pierre-niney-qui-fait-le-proces-du-sexisme_143606.html> [accessed 25 August 2022].

Chrisafis, Angelique. *France Falls Out of Love with Topless Sunbathing* (2009), *The Guardian* <https://amp.theguardian.com/lifeandstyle/2009/jul/22/topless-bathing-france> [accessed 16 July 2022].

——. *French PM Suggests Naked Breasts Represent France Better than a Headscarf* (2016), *The Guardian* <https://amp.theguardian.com/world/2016/aug/30/france-manuel-valls-breasts-headscarf-burkini-ban-row> [accessed 10 July 2022].

CNEWS. 'Hijab, voile, Burqa : de quoi parle-t-on et que dit la loi ?' (2021), *CNews*, <https://www.cnews.fr/france/2021-11-03/hijab-voile-burqa-de-quoi-parle-t-et-que-dit-la-loi-737077> [accessed 8 August 2023].

Cooper, Glenda. *Women Too Scared to Go Out Alone* (1997), *Independent* <https://www.independent.co.uk/news/uk/home-news/women-too-scared-to-go-out-alone-1273125.html> [accessed 7 September 2022].

Cooper, Robin and Bruce Lilyea. 'I'm Interested in Autoethnography, but How Do I Do It?', *The Qualitative Report* (2022). PDF.

CSA. *Le catholicisme en France* (2013), Archive.org. Available at: <http:/ www.csa.eu/multimedia/data/etudes/etudes/etu20130329-note-d-anal yse-csa-decrypte-mars-2013.pdf> [accessed 21 September 2022].

Das, Shanti. *Inside the Violent, Misogynistic World of TikTok's New Star, Andrew Tate* (2022), *The Guardian* <https://amp.theguardian.com/technology/2022/aug/06/andrew-tate-violent-misogynistic-world-of-tiktok-new-star> [accessed 22 August 2022].

Davey, Melissa. *Online Violence against Women 'Flourishing', and Most Common on Facebook, Survey Finds* (2020), *The Guardian* <https://amp.theguardian.com/ society/2020/oct/05/online-violence-against-women-flourishing-and-most-common-on-facebook-survey-finds> [accessed 19 August 2022].

Delphy, Christine, and Diana Leonard. *Que veut dire « le privé est politique »* ? (2019), *Lmsi.net* <https://lmsi.net/Que-veut-dire-le-prive-est-politique-3> [accessed 25 July 2022].

Drouelle, Léa. *Wonderbra tente une pub 'féministe' et se fait tacler* (2018), *Terrafemina* <https://www.terrafemina.com/article/sexisme-la-nouvelle-pub-wonderbra-fait-reagir_a347053/1> [accessed 7 August 2022].

Dylan, Lady. *Je veux comprendre … le slut-shaming* (2017), *Madmoizelle* <https:// www.madmoizelle.com/slut-shaming-115244> [accessed 8 September 2022].

El Euldj, Manal Lyna, and Ambre Marionneau. *'Expose-toi et tais-toi' : les femmes, premières victimes des réseaux sociaux* (2020), *Numerique-investigation. org* <https://numerique-investigation.org/la-critique-systematique-des-personnes-percues-comme-femme-sur-les-reseaux-sociaux/4847/> [accessed 22 August 2022].

Everhart, Ruth. *Who's Responsible for the Male Gaze?* (2021), *Ruth Everhart* <https:// rutheverhart.com/stewart-allen-clark-preacher-whos-responsible-for-the-male-gaze/> [accessed 11 July 2022].

Fisk, Catriona. *A Decent Woman? The Breastfeeding and Visibility Debate Is Nothing New* (2016), *The Conversation* <http://theconversation.com/a-decent-woman-the-breastfeeding-and-visibility-debate-is-nothing-new-57728> [accessed 30 June 2022].

Foucher, Matthieu. *Où en sont les études de genre en France ?* (2019), *Les Inrocks* <https://www.lesinrocks.com/actu/ou-en-sont-les-etudes-de-genre-en-fra nce-180570-12-09-2019/> [accessed 26 September 2022]

Gaillard, Claire-Lise. *Jean-Claude Bologne Histoire de la pudeur* (n.d.), *Sentiment et modernité* <https://sentiment.hypotheses.org/84> [accessed 18 September 2022].

Galouise, Pierre. *Top 10 des magazines pour ado des années 2000 (ceux qui nous ont le plus structuré intellectuellement)* (2021), *Topito* <https://www.topito.com/top-magazine-people-2000> [accessed 10 September 2022].

Global Trends in Religiosity and Atheism 1980 to 2020 (2020), *Colin Mathers* <https://colinmathers.com/2020/09/30/global-trends-in-religiosity-and-atheism-1980-to-2020/> [accessed 12 July 2022].

Groskop, Viv. *Not Your Mother's Milk* (2007), *The Guardian* <https://amp.theg uardian.com/society/2007/jan/05/health.medicineandhealth> [accessed 29 June 2022].

Guedj, Léa. *Dans les collèges et les lycées, tenue correcte exigée … surtout pour les filles*, (2018), *France Inter* <https://www.radiofrance.fr/franceinter/dans-les-colle ges-et-les-lycees-tenue-correcte-exigee-surtout-pour-les-filles-9176333> [accessed 10 September 2022].

Hamou, Cynthia. *Les seins et leurs complexes : forme, taille et harmonie* (2019), *Chirurgien esthétique femme à Grenoble – Rhône Alpes* <https://doct eur-hamou.com/seins-leurs-complexes-forme-taille-harmonie> [accessed 8 August 2022].

Harris, Danielle. *Sexist Censorship on Social Media* (2016), *The DePaulia*. Available at: <https://depauliaonline.com/19576/opinions/censorship-free-the-nipple/ > [accessed 19 August 2022].

Harrison, Virginia. *Outrage Erupts over Facebook's Decision on Graphic Videos* (2013), *CNNMoney* <https://money.cnn.com/2013/10/22/news/companies/faceb ook-violent-videos/> [accessed 7 September 2022].

Ho, Geoff. *Wonderbra: Hello Sexism, Cry Feminists* (2018), *Daily Express* <https:// www.express.co.uk/life-style/life/1053249/wonderbra-adverts-hello-boys-sex ism-feminism> [accessed 16 July 2022].

Hunt, Amy. *Is It Bad Not to Wear a Bra? Here's the Lowdown on What Could Happen to Your Cleavage* (2020), *Woman and Home Magazine* <https://www.woman andhome.com/health-and-wellbeing/bra-health-boobs-posture-354096/> [accessed 7 August 2022].

Hussonnois-Alaya, Céline. « *On doit se cacher »: l'allaitement en public est-il encore tabou?* (2021), *BFMTV* <https://www.bfmtv.com/societe/on-doit-se-cacher- l-allaitement-en-public-est-il-encore-tabou_AN-202110030005.html> [accessed 30 June 2022].

Ide, Sémiramis. *Le dico des filles, le top du sexisme* (2014), *Information TV5MONDE* <https://information.tv5monde.com/terriennes/le-dico-des-filles-le-top-du- sexisme-3126> [accessed 13 September 2022].

Inman, Nick. *The Complex History of Love, Sex and the French* (2021), <https:// www.connexionfrance.com> <https://www.connexionfrance.com/article/ Mag/Culture/The-complex-history-of-love-sex-and-the-French> [accessed 15 September 2022].

Johnson, Bysoraya. *The Problem with 'Pick Me' Girls* (2020), *Affinitymagazine.Us* <http://affinitymagazine.us/2020/06/25/the-problem-with-pick-me-girls/> [accessed 9 September 2022].

Jones, Christopher P. *Why the Virgin Mary's Bare Breast Caused a Problem for Artists* (2022), *Thinksheet* <https://medium.com/thinksheet/the-artistic-problem- with-the-virgin-marys-bare-breast-19e3d4339008> [accessed 9 July 2022].

Kelly, Emma. *Addressing Rape Culture : The Unbearable Flippancy of French Media* (2022), *Institut Du Genre En Géopolitique* <https://igg-geo.org/?p= 8230&lang=en> [accessed 4 August 2023].

——. *Andrew Tate Claims Women Should 'Bear Responsibility' for Being Raped* (2017), *Metro.co.uk* <https://metro.co.uk/2017/10/19/big-brothers-andrew-tate-says-women-should-bear-responsibility-for-being-raped-in-vile-tweets-7011756/> [accessed 22 August 2022].

——. *Andrew Tate: Money-Making Scheme for Fans of 'Extreme Misogynist' Closes* (2022), *The Guardian* <https://amp.theguardian.com/media/2022/aug/20/ andrew-tate-money-making-scheme-for-fans-of-extreme-misogynist-closes> [accessed 22 August 2022].

Kraus, François and Louise Jussian. *Pour les français, qu'est ce qu'une "tenue correcte" pour une fille au lycée?* (2020), Ifop.com <https:// www.ifop.com/ wp- cont ent/ uplo ads/ 2020/ 09/ Ifop_ C rop_ mar.top_ 2 020.09.23.pdf> [accessed 10 September 2022].

Laffut, Florence, and Florence Ronveaux. *Slut-shaming : un nouveau phénomène vieux comme le monde* (2014), *CVFE – Dire NON aux violences conjugales !* <https:// www.cvfe.be/publications/analyses/227-slut-shaming-un-nouveau-phenom ene-vieux-comme-le-monde> [accessed 9 September 2022].

Le boom du « No Bra », tendance de fond ou effet de mode ? (2020), *IFOP,* <https:// www.ifop.com/publication/le-boom-du-no-bra-tendance-de-fond-ou-effet-de-mode/> [accessed 12 July 2022].

Le Dico des filles : rose toxique (2014), *Gazette des femmes* <https://gazettedesfem mes.ca/9813/le-dico-des-filles-rose-toxique/> [accessed 10 September 2022].

Lingerie Industry Reports: Statistics, Trend, Analysis & Market Research (n.d.), *Reportlinker.com* <https://www.reportlinker.com/ci02123/Underwear. html>[accessed 8 August 2022].

A Look at the Evolution of Lingerie Ads (2016), *Bra Doctor's Blog | Now That's Lingerie* <https://blog.nowthatslingerie.com/lingerie-2/a-look-at-the-evolut ion-of-lingerie-ads/2016/08/08> [accessed 8 August 2022].

Ma copine se met trop en valeur sur insta (n.d.), *Jeuxvideo.com* <https://www.jeuxvi deo.com/forums/42-51-59198062-2-0-1-0-ma-copine-se-met-trop-en-valeur-sur-insta.htm> [accessed 25 July 2022].

Ma copine veut faire un insta 'fitness girl' (n.d.), *Jeuxvideo.com* <https://www.jeuxvi deo.com/forums/42-78-47211584-2-0-1-0-ma-copine-veut-faire-un-insta-fitn ess-girl.htm> [accessed 25 July 2022].

Maguire, Moira and Brid Delahunt. 'Doing a Thematic Analysis: A Practical, Step-by-Step Guide for Learning and Teaching Scholars'. *All Ireland Journal of*

Higher Education 9, no. 3 (2017), <https://ojs.aishe.org/index.php/aishe-j/arti
cle/view/335> [accessed 15 September 2022].

Manning, Charles. *Nicki Minaj Worries about the Impact She Has Had on Young
Women* (2018), *Daily Front Row*. Available at: <https://fashionweekdaily.
com/nikki-minaj-elle-cover/> [accessed 25 August 2022].

Mark, Joshua J. *Women in the Middle Ages* (2019), *World History Encyclopedia*.
<https://www.worldhistory.org/article/1345/women-in-the-middle-ages/>
[accessed 12 July 2022].

Martin, Delphine. *Le soutien-gorge : une invention bourguignonne* (2018), *France
Bleu*   <https://www.francebleu.fr/infos/societe/le-soutien-gorge-une-invent
ion-bourguignonne-1520016016> [accessed 8 August 2022].

Marty, Barbara. *À l'origine du soutien-gorge : une féministe révolutionnaire*
(2020), *France Culture* <https://www.radiofrance.fr/franceculture/a-l-orig
ine-du-soutien-gorge-une-feministe-revolutionnaire-1187756> [accessed   15
July 2022].

Menez, Lydia, Margaux Ravard, and Auriane Guerithault. *« On culpabilise les
jeunes filles dans tout l'ouvrage » : la rédaction a relu le « Dico des filles »*
(2022), *ELLE* <https://www.elle.fr/Societe/News/On-culpabilise-les-jeunes-
filles-dans-tout-l-ouvrage-la-redaction-a-relu-le-Dico-des-filles-4021909> [ac-
cessed 10 September 2022].

Meyer, Mati. *Art: Representation of Biblical Women* (n.d.), *Jewish Women's Archive*.
<https://jwa.org/encyclopedia/article/art-representation-of-biblical-
women> [accessed 12 July 2022].

The New York Times. *Will Instagram ever 'free the nipple'?* (2019), *The New York
Times*. Available at: <https://www.nytimes.com/2019/11/22/arts/design/
instagram-free-the-nipple.html> [accessed 19 August 2022].

Nikon Camera Ad: Bigger Is Better – Sociological Images (2009), *Thesocietypages.
org* <https://thesocietypages.org/socimages/2009/05/08/nikon-camera-ad-
bigger-is-better/> [accessed 8 August 2022].

Ortiz-Ospina, Esteban. *The Rise of Social Media* (2019), *Our World in Data* <https://
ourworldindata.org/rise-of-social-media> [accessed 7 September 2022].

Papadopoulos, Linda. *Sexualisation of Young People – Review* [eBook] (2010),
Available   at: <https://dera.ioe.ac.uk/10738/1/sexualisation-young-people.
pdf> [accessed 26 August 2022].

Peguy, Olivier. *#MeToo, #Balancetonporc, trois ans après* (2020), *Euronews*. Available
at: <https://fr.euronews.com/2020/10/21/metoo-balancetonporc-trois-ans-
apres> [accessed 25 August 2022].

Planetoscope – Statistiques : Consommation de Lingerie En France (2018), *Planetoscope.
com*   <https://www.planetoscope.com/lamour/1762-consommation-de-linge
rie-en-france.html> [accessed 8 August 2022].

Population française selon la religion France (2020), *Statista* <https://fr.statista.com/statistiques/472017/population-religion-france/> [accessed 12 July 2022]

Promulgation de La Loi Relative à La Séparation Des Églises et de l'État (2016), *Gouvernement.Fr*, <https://www.gouvernement.fr/partage/8764-le-9-decembre-1905-est-promulguee-la-loi-%20relative-à-la-séparation-des-Églises-et-de-l-État> [accessed 12 July 2022].

Pruitt, Sarah. *What Are the Four Waves of Feminism?* (2022), *History* <https://www.history.com/news/feminism-four-waves> [accessed 18 August 2022].

Rebufa, Bérénice. *Dim fait complexer les ados avec un soutien-gorge qui 'gomme les imperfections'* (2016), *Konbini* <https://www.konbini.com/archive/dim-encore-soutien-gorge/> [accessed 7 August 2022].

Rosenfield, Kat. *What's Wrong with Lingerie?* (2021), *UnHerd* <https://unherd.com/2021/06/whats-wrong-with-lingerie/> [accessed 30 July 2022].

Rosser, Kristen. *Christianity and the 'Male Gaze'* (2013), *Wordgazer's Words* <http://krwordgazer.blogspot.com/2013/07/christianity-and-male-gaze.html> [accessed 11 July 2022].

Sieczkowski, Cavan. *Pat Robertson Blames 'Awful Looking' Women for Marital Problems* (2013), *HuffPost UK* <https://www.huffpost.com/entry/pat-robertson-blames-awful-looking-women-marriage-problems_n_2479459> [accessed 11 July 2022].

Slate. *The Tragic Story behind Victoria's Secret* (2013), *HuffPost* <https://www.huffpost.com/entry/victorias-secret_n_4181683> [accessed 30 July 2022].

Slut-shaming », exhibitionnisme : les réseaux sociaux bouleversent la vie des adolescentes (2016), *L'Obs*. Available at: <https://www.nouvelobs.com/rue89/rue89-sur-les-reseaux/20160303.RUE2341/slut-shaming-exhibitionnisme-les-reseaux-sociaux-bouleversent-la-vie-des-adolescentes.html> [accessed 26 August 2022].

Sparks, Hannah. *Pastor Slammed for Telling Wives to 'Lose Weight,' Look Less 'Butch'* (2021), *New York Post* <https://nypost.com/2021/03/03/pastor-slammed-for-telling-wives-to-lose-weight-look-less-butch/> [accessed 11 July 2022].

Spencer-Elliott, Lydia. *This Is the Story behind Janet Jackson's Super Bowl 'Wardrobe Malfunction'* (2022), *Grazia* <https://graziadaily.co.uk/life/tv-and-film/janet-jackson-documentary-timberlake-super-bowl/> [accessed 19 August 2022].

Suarez, Sonia. *Objectification and Women Empowerment: The Social Media Scene* (2021), *Engagewithscience.org* <https://engagewithscience.org/objectification-and-women-empowerment-the-social-media-scene/> [accessed 18 August 2022].

Topi, Ana. *The First Bra in History of Herminie Cadolle 1898* (2018), *Runway Magazine* <https://runwaymagazines.com/the-first-bra-in-history-of-herminie-cadolle-1898/> [accessed 25 July 2022].

Torgemen, Émilie. *Pourquoi les Françaises sont de moins en moins adeptes du topless* (2019), *Le Parisien* <https://www.leparisien.fr/societe/pourquoi-les-francai ses-sont-de-moins-en-moins-adeptes-du-topless-24-07-2019-8122524.php> [accessed 11 August 2022].

The Use of Misogynistic Terms on Twitter (2016), *Demos.co.uk* <https://www.demos. co.uk/wp-content/uploads/2016/05/Misogyny-online.pdf> [accessed 9 September 2022].

Wade, Mike. *Social Media Fuels Offline Misogyny, Says Top Lawyer* (2022), *Times* <https://www.thetimes.co.uk/article/social-media-fuels-offl ine-misogyny-says-top-lawyer-qcpnd68sq> [accessed 22 August 2022].

What Is Hypersexualization (n.d.), *Igi-global.com* <https://www.igi-global.com/dic tionary/overcoming-barriers/94467> [accessed 18 August 2022].

What Is Purity Culture? (2019), *Linda Kay Klein* <https://lindakayklein.com/what-is-purity-culture/> [accessed 12 July 2022].

Academic articles

Armstrong, Elizabeth A., Laura T. Hamilton, Elizabeth M. Armstrong, and J. Lotus Seeley. '"Good Girls": Gender, Social Class, and Slut Discourse on Campus'. *Social Psychology Quarterly* 77, no. 2 (2014): 100–22.

Baxter, Alyssa. 'Faux Activism in Recent Female-Empowering Advertising'. *Elon Journal of Undergraduate Research in Communications* 6, no. 1 (2015). <http:// www.inquiriesjournal.com/articles/1133/faux-activism-in-recent-female-emp owering-advertising> [accessed 8 August 2022].

Blum, R. W., K. Mmari, and C. Moreau. 'It Begins at 10: How Gender Expectations Shape Early Adolescence around the World' [online]. *The Journal of Adolescent Health: Official Publication of the Society for Adolescent Medicine* 61, 4 Suppl. (2017): S3–S4. Available at: <https://www.jahonline.org/article/S1054-139X(17)30355-5/fulltext> [accessed 20 September 2022].

Brodie, Ian. '"The Harsh Reality of Being a Woman": First Bra Experiences'. *Ethnologies* 29, no. 1–2 (2008): 81–106.

Daniels, Elizabeth A., Eileen L. Zurbriggen, and L. Monique Ward. 'Becoming an Object: A Review of Self-Objectification in Girls'. *Body Image* 33 (2020): 278–99.

De Kuyper, Eric. 'The Freudian Construction of Sexuality: The Gay Foundations of Heterosexuality and Straight Homophobia'. *Journal of Homosexuality* 24, no. 3–4 (1993): 137–44.

De Rasse, Marie. 'Vêtement féminin et pudeur. L'exemple parisien, XIVe–XVe siècles'. *Hypothèses* 13, no. 1 (2010): 119–28.

Dolezal, Luna. 'The (in)Visible Body: Feminism, Phenomenology, and the Case of Cosmetic Surgery'. *Hypatia* 25, no. 2 (2010): 357–75.

Favre, Camille. 'The Pin-Up: American Eroticism and Patriotism during the Second World War'. *Inflexions* 38, no. 2 (2018): 181.

Gonzalez-Quijano, Lola. 'Bologne Jean-Claude, Pudeurs féminines. Voilées, dévoilées, révélées' (2011), *Genre sexualité & société* <https://journals.openedit ion.org/gss/1918> [accessed 18 September 2022].

Granger, Kristen L., Laura D. Hanish, Olga Kornienko, and et al. 'Preschool Teachers' Facilitation of Gender-Typed and Gender-Neutral Activities during Free Play'. *Sex Roles* 76, no. 7–8 (2017): 498–510.

Hammarberg, K., M. Kirkman, and S. de Lacey. 'Qualitative Research Methods: When to Use Them and How to Judge Them'. *Human Reproduction (Oxford, England)* 31, no. 3 (2016): 498–501.

Harlow, Daniel. 'Creation According to Genesis: Literary Genre, Cultural Context, Theological Truth'. *Christian Scholar's Review* 37, no. 2 (n.d.): 163–98.

Iacovidou, Nicoletta. 'Breastfeeding in Public: A Global Review of Different Attitudes towards It'. *Journal of Paediatrics & Neonatal Care* 1, no. 6 (2014).

Jacklin, C. N., J. A. DiPietro, and E. E. Maccoby. 'Sex-Typing Behavior and Sex-Typing Pressure in Child/Parent Interaction' [online]. *Archives of Sexual Behavior* 13, no. 5 (1984): 413–25.

Jewell, J., C. Spears Brown, and B. Perry. 'All My Friends Are Doing It: Potentially Offensive Sexual Behavior Perpetration within Adolescent Social Networks' [online]. *Journal of Research on Adolescence: The Official Journal of the Society for Research on Adolescence* 25, no. 3 (2015): 592–604.

Kelly, Moira. 'The Role of Theory in Qualitative Health Research'. *Family Practice* 27, no. 3 (2010): 285–90.

King, Angela. 'The Prisoner of Gender: Foucault and the Disciplining of the Female Body'. *Journal of International Women's Studies* 5 (2004): 29–39.

Lieber, Marylène. 'Le sentiment d'insécurité des femmes dans l'espace public : une entrave à la citoyenneté ?'. *Nouvelles questions féministes* 21, no. 1 (2002): 41–56.

Liotard, Philippe, and Sandrine Jamain-Samson. 'La « Lolita » et la « sex bomb », figures de socialisation des jeunes filles. L'hypersexualisation en question'. *Sociologie et sociétés* 43, no. 1 (2011): 45–71.

Lussier, Judith. *Un symbole d'oppression* (2019), *Journal Métro* <https://journalme tro.com/actualites/national/2302827/un-symbole-doppression/> [accessed 16 July 2022].

Manning, Jimmie. 'Paradoxes of (Im)Purity: Affirming Heteronormativity and Queering Heterosexuality in Family Discourses of Purity Pledges'. *Women's Studies in Communication* 38, no. 1 (2015): 99–117.

Mardon, Aurélia. 'Les femmes et la lingerie : Intimité corporelle et morale sexuelle'. *Champ psychosomatique* 27, no. 3 (2002): 69.

Means, Kira K. *'Not Like Other Girls*: Implicit and Explicit Dimensions of Internalized Sexism and Behavioral Outcomes', WWU Graduate School Collection (2021).

Millsted, Rachel and Hannah Frith. 'Being Large-Breasted: Women Negotiating Embodiment'. *Women's Studies International Forum* 26, no. 5 (2003): 455–65.

Mol, Sophie. *Le slut-shaming, cet inconnu qui vous veut du bien ?* (2017), *Uclouvain. be.* Available at: <https://dial.uclouvain.be/memoire/ucl/en/object/the sis%3A10875/datastream/PDF_01/view> [accessed 8 September 2022].

Moradi, Bonnie and Yu-Ping Huang. 'Objectification Theory and Psychology of Women: A Decade of Advances and Future Directions'. *Psychology of Women Quarterly* 32, no. 4 (2008): 377–98.

Mummey, Kevin, and Kathryn Reyerson. 'Whose City Is This? Hucksters, Domestic Servants, Wet-Nurses, Prostitutes, and Slaves in Late Medieval Western Mediterranean Urban Society: Whose City Is This?'. *History Compass* 9, no. 12 (2011): 910–22.

Papp, Leanna J., Mindy J. Erchull, Miriam Liss, et al. 'Slut-Shaming on Facebook: Do Social Class or Clothing Affect Perceived Acceptability?'. *Gender Issues* 34, no. 3 (2017): 240–57.

Ponterotto, Diane. 'Resisting the Male Gaze: Feminist Responses to the "Normatization" of the Female Body in Western Culture'. *Journal of International Women's Studies* 17, no. 1 (2016): 133–51.

Quemener, Nelly. '« Ma Chérie, Il Faut Révéler Ta Féminité ! »: Rhétorique Du Choix et de L'émancipation Dans Les Émissions de Relooking En France'. *Raisons Politiques* 62, no. 2 (2016): 35.

Richardson, Laurel, and Susan Brownmiller. 'Femininity'. *Contemporary Sociology* 14, no. 1 (1985): 80.

Riordan, Jan, and Betty Ann Countryman. 'Part I: Infant Feeding Patterns Past and Present'. *JOGN Nursing; Journal of Obstetric, Gynaecologic, and Neonatal Nursing* 9, no. 4 (1980).

Smith, Dorothy E. et al. *7 Feminist and Gender Theories*, Sagepub.com. Available at: <https://www.sagepub.com/sites/default/files/upm-binaries/38628_7.pdf> [accessed 16 August 2022].

Stevens, Emily E., Thelma E. Patrick, and Rita Pickler. 'A History of Infant Feeding'. *The Journal of Perinatal Education* 18, no. 2 (2009): 32–9.

Van der Putten, Jan. 'Negotiating the Great Depression: The Rise of Popular Culture and Consumerism in Early-1930s Malaya'. *Journal of Southeast Asian Studies* 1 (2010): 21–45.

Wood, Rachel. '"You Do Act Differently When You're in It": Lingerie and Femininity'. *Journal of Gender Studies* 25, no. 1 (2016): 10–23.

Zaikman, Yuliana, and Amy E. Houlihan. 'It's Just a Breast: An Examination of the Effects of Sexualization, Sexism, and Breastfeeding Familiarity on Evaluations of Public Breastfeeding'. *BMC Pregnancy and Childbirth* 22, no. 1 (2022): 122.

Zancarini-Fournel, Michelle. 'Genre et politique : les années 1968'. *Vingtième siècle* 75, no. 3 (2002): 133.

Book chapters

De Beauvoir, Simone. *The Second Sex* (New York: Knopf, 1953), 189–90.

Freud, Sigmund. 'Female Sexuality'. In *The Future of an Illusion, Civilization and Its Discontents, and Other Works* (1931), 221–44.

Jackson, Sue, and Tina Vares. 'Media "Sluts": "Tween" Girls' Negotiations of Postfeminist Sexual Subjectivities in Popular Culture'. In *New Femininities*, edited by C. Scharff, & R. Gill (London: Palgrave Macmillan UK, 2011), 134–46.

Lee Bartky, Sandra. 'Foucault, Femininity, and the Modernization of Patriarchal Power'. In *Femininity and Domination* (Routledge, 2015), 73–92.

Mulvey, Laura. (ed.). 'Visual Pleasure and Narrative Cinema'. In *Visual and Other Pleasures* (2nd ed.) (Houndmills, Basingstoke, Hampshire, England/ New York: Palgrave Macmillan 2009), 14–30.

O'Reilly, Andrea. 'Wet Nursing'. In *Encyclopaedia of Motherhood*, edited by Andrea O'Reilly (Thousand Oaks, CA: SAGE Publications, Inc., 2010), 1272–73.

Pitts-Taylor, Victoria. (ed.). 'Cultural History of the Breast'. In *Cultural Encyclopaedia of the Body [2 Volumes]*, edited by Pitts-Taylor (Westport, CT: Greenwood Press, 2008).

Ringrose, Jessica. 'Are You Sexy, Flirty, or a Slut? Exploring "Sexualization" and How Teen Girls Perform/Negotiate Digital Sexual Identity on Social Networking Sites'. In *New Femininities*, edited by C. Scharff, & R. Gill (London: Palgrave Macmillan UK, 2011), 99–116.

Winch, Alison. 'The Girlfriend Gaze'. In *Girlfriends and Postfeminist Sisterhood* (London: Palgrave Macmillan UK, 2013), 8–32, 22.

Books

Bateman, Victoria. *Naked Feminism: Breaking the Cult of Female Modesty* (Oxford: Polity Press, 2023).

The Bible. *New International Version* (1 Timothy 2:9–15).

Boutin-Arnaud, Marie-Noël, and Sandrine Tasmadjian. *Le vêtement* (Paris: Éditions Nathan, 1997).

Brooks Gardner, Carol. *Passing by: Gender and Public Harassment* (Berkeley, CA: University of California Press, 1995).

Craig, Maxine. *Ain't I a Beauty Queen?: Culture, Social Movements, and the Politics of Race* (New York: Oxford University Press, 2002).

Davis, Dána-Ain and Christa Craven. *Feminist Ethnography: Thinking Through Methodologies, Challenges, and Possibilities* (Lanham, Maryland: Rowman & Littlefield, 2016).

Farrell-Beck, Jane, and Colleen Gau. *Uplift: The Bra in America* (Baltimore, MD: University of Pennsylvania Press, 2001).

Fields, Jill. *An Intimate Affair Women, Lingerie, and Sexuality* (Berkeley: University of California Press, 2007).

Friedman, Jaclyn. *What You Really Really Want: The Smart Girl's Shame-Free Guide to Sex and Safety* (Seattle, WA: Seal Press, 2011).

Kaiser, Susan B., and Denise N. Green. *Fashion and Cultural Studies* (London, England: Bloomsbury Visual Arts, 2021).

Lee, Shayne. *Erotic Revolutionaries: Black Women, Sexuality, and Popular Culture* (Lanham, MD: Hamilton Books, 2010).

McCormack, Catherine, *Women in the Picture: Women, Art and the Power of Looking* (Basingstoke, England: Icon Books, 2021).

Mitchell, Juliet. *Psychoanalysis and Feminism*, 2nd ed. (Harlow, England: Penguin Books, 2000).

Pratt, Mary Louise. *Imperial Eyes: Travel Writing and Transculturation* (London and New York: Routledge, 1992).

Sprague, Joey. *Feminist Methodologies for Critical Researchers: Bridging Differences*, 2nd ed. (New York: Rowman & Littlefield, 2016).

Tarlo, Emma. *Visibly Muslim: Fashion, Politics, Faith* (London, England: Bloomsbury Academic, 2010).

Filmography

'Emily in Paris', Netflix, 2020, episode 3, season 1.

Index

www.ingramcontent.com/pod-product-compliance
Lightning Source LLC
Chambersburg PA
CBHW050535270326
41926CB00015B/3232